HEALTH AND ENVIRONMENT

Encyclopaedia of Environmental Pollution and Awareness in 21st Century Series

HEALTH AND ENVIRONMENT

Edited by

V.K. Prabhakar

ANMOL PUBLICATIONS PVT. LTD.

NEW DELHI - 110 002 (INDIA)

ANMOL PUBLICATIONS PVT. LTD.
4374/4B, Ansari Road, Daryaganj
New Delhi - 110 002

Health and Environment

First Edition, 2001
ISBN 81-261-0907-6

PRINTED IN INDIA

Published by J.L. Kumar for Anmol Publications Pvt. Ltd., New Delhi - 110 002 and Printed at Mehra Offset Press, Delhi.

Contents

PREFACE

Today, the cry of 'pollution' is heard from all the nooks and corners of the world, and pollution has become a major threat to the very existence of mankind on this earth. It is the major challenge of our times.

The pollution of various resources has gone to such an extent that we are unable to breathe fresh air and drink fresh water. On one hand the advancements of science and technology have added to the human comforts by giving us automobiles, electrical appliances, supersonic jets, space crafts, better medicines, better chemicals to control harmful insects and other pests, etc., but, on the other hand, they have given us a very serious problem to face that is pollution. Pollution can be defined as an undesirable change in the physical, chemical, or biological characteristics of the air, water, or land that can harmfully affect health, survival, or activities of humans or other living organisms.

Pollution does not have to cause physical harm, but it may merely interfere with human activities. Chemicals spewed into the air or water from an industrial plant may be harmful to humans and other organisms living near the plant. If expensive pollution controls are required, the plant may be forced to shut down.

India faces serious problems of environmental pollution. Water pollution from untreated community and industrial wastes flowing into our rivers and streams, increasing use of fertilizers and pesticides, dumping of organic wastes etc., are issues that need to be tackled on the priority. Air pollution, long regarded as the bane of industrialised nations looms large over our country.

Here, we are presenting this *Encyclopaedia of Environmental Pollution and Awareness in Twenty-first Century* in fifty volumes with a view to make people conscious about the seriousness of pollution in the present time and its remedies.

Editor

1 INTRODUCTION

Environmental health is that aspect of public health that is concerned with those forms of life substances, forces and conditions in the surroundings of man that may exert an influence on man's health and well-being. This definition includes other people as part of man's surroundings that contribute to the status of environmental health.

Early definitions of public health reflected concern with communicable disease and stressed prevention of disease. While prevention of undesirable conditions and consequences is fundamental to most definitions, public health, or just plain health, today has a much broader connotation including the attainment of desirable positive health values, in addition to the prevention of undesired negative ones.

Consequently, the definition of public health developed by the World Health Organization, and widely accepted states. "Health is a state of complete physical, mental, and social well-being and not merely the absence of disease or infirmity." In recent years, environmental engineering is a term that has come into wide use. While the meaning of this terminology is some what controversial is some circles, it generally refers to the study of man-environment inter-relationships and the modification of the environment for man's benefit. To the extent that there is concern for man's environment as it relates from illness, health maintenance, human efficiency, comfort and the enjoyment of life, use of property, and management of resources. At times, it becomes impossible and useless, because of direct and indirect interrelationships, to make any distinction between those activities concerned with man's health and other aspects of environmental engineering and science, as in air and water pollution. Both natural and social sciences have application in the development of a suitable environment for man.

"Sanitation is a way of life' according to the National Sanitation Foundation, Frequently, throughout history, the status of the environment, which historically has been equated with sanitation but is now much broader in concept, has been the measure of civilization. In fact, the aggregation of population has always seemed to create environmental health problems which had to be solved before the populace could survive and enlarge. The earliest public health measures were concerned with environmental matters.

Many customs, taboos, and religious practices has their roots in observed or presumed interaction between man and environmental conditions. Moses 'Law has dictates concerning sanitation which could have applications today. The supply of water and the removal of wastes have been critical problems for aggregations of people. Drainage systems were built by the Minoans (3000 - 1500 B.C.), and the Egyptians (1000 B.C.) were noted for irrigation and other public health measure. The Grecians were concerned about personal hygiene and cleanliness.

The Romans built aqueducts and drainage systems which were marvels. Archaeological excavations in India and the Middle East show that other ancient civilizations had similar systems, although not as impressive as those in Rome. In the Middle Ages, there began a change in social organization which initiated the rise of many cities, with the growth of these cities, diseases were more easily communicated from one person to another. Terrible pandemics swept through the cities of Europe, decimating the population. Such diseases as cholera, associated with polluted water, and bulonic plague (the "black death"), associated with rats, were rampant. The very existence of the cities was threatened.

With the Renaissance and the development of the miscroscope, it became possible to identify the bacteria that caused communicable diseases. The first depiction of bacteria was by Anthony van Leeuwenhoek in 1683. Through the work of Pasteur, Koch, and others knowledge of the role of bacteria as a cause of disease was developed and enlarged. Interestingly, the earliest applications of Pasteur's work had commercial values in fermentation and animal disease. (In modern times, the American public was seemingly unconcerned about trichinosis being spread by the feeding of uncooked garbage to swine, but when a disease of hogs, vesicular exanthema, was found to be transmitted thereby, laws prohibiting the practice were passed with great speed).

Before science established the cause of disease, man had, at times, instinctively avoided circumstances suspected of causing disease. Thus an epidemic of cholera and typhoid on London in 1854 was terminated by the simple expedient of removing the handle to a pump on a well located adjacent to a sewer. The term "malaria" was the name applied to a disease thought to be associated with bad air, which was equated to the night air. We now know, of course, that the female anopheles mosquito attacks man and transmits the causative organism. Unfortunately, many of todays environmental hazards have been introduced so rapidly that man's instinctive reaction have not had time to adapt so he is not aware of their dangers. Nevertheless, such designations as "New Oriens" or "Yokohama" asthama, may well be the same intuitive labeling, witness "miners consumption" later found to be silicosis. With the coming of the Industrial Revolution new hazards to man were introduced into his environment-physical injury from machines and work methods, toxic exposures, and other stresses. It was about this time that the first organization of public resources and society in the interest of public health began.

Developments in England and the United States were somewhat parallel. Although they did not result in immediate achievements, in both cases social organization for public health can be traced to two reports. In England it was the "Report on an Inquiry into the Sanitary Conditions of the Labouring Population of Great Britain" by Edwin Chadwick in 1842. Chadwick's report revealed that one-half the children of the labouring population died before their fifth birthday.

At that time he found that, in some cities, the average age at death was 36 for gentry, 22 for tradesmen and 16 for labours. Chadwick became interested in health as it related to poverty, and he was Secretary of the Poor Law Commissioners at the time of his investigations and report.

In 1850 in the United States, the "Report of the Sanitary Commission of Massachusetts" was published. Lemuel Shatuck, a bookseller who became interested in statistics, was head of the commission. These two reports are hailed today as historical landmarks, not so much because they were forerunners of actions ultimately taken to establish organized public health agencies, but because of their insights and perspectives.

In Shatuck's report, we read the following:

> We recommend that provision be made for obtaining observations of the atmospheric phenomena, on a systematic and uniform plan, at different stations in the Commonwealth...
>
> We recommend that measures be taken to prevent as far as practicable, the smoke nuisance....
>
> (Noting that)...the tendency of our people seems to be toward social concentration...(this report continues):

We recommend that in laying out new towns and villages, and in extending those already laid our, ample provision be made for a supply, in purity and abundance, of light, air, and water; for drainage and sewerage, for paving and for cleanliness.

Additional recommendations related to housing, schools, occupational health, and adulterated food and drugs. The report also urged..." that person be specially educated in sanitary science..." Now, over 100 years later, these environmental problems continue to plague us and in some instances, are intensified.

The status of man's health represents the result of complex interactions between his internal biological system and the total external environmental system. This text is concerned primarily with the external environmental system, but it should be obvious that the interactions between the environment and man's biological system must always be before us. The environment is both natural and modified by man's work and presence. The element of the environmental system of concern are diagrammed in Fig. 1.

Man as a biological organism has developed in an environment which is being changed more rapidly than ever before. These changes may tax his adaptive capacities. Even where the adapts, we are not certain what the costs to his biological system may be. Certain environmental conditions are necessary to sustain life. Still other affect body functions, performance, and comfort, air, water, food and shelter are requirements for man's survival.

Life support	*Man's Activities*	*Residues and Wastes*
Air	Home	Solids
Water	Work	Liquids
Shelter	Transportation	Gases

Environmental Hazards

Biological	*Chemical*	*Physical*	*Psychological*	*Sociological*
Animal	Poisons and	Vibration	Stress	Overcrowding
Insect	Toxins	Radiation	Boredom	Isolation
Microbiolo-gical	Irritants	Forces & Abrasion	Discomfort	Anomie
			Depression	
		Humidity		

Fig 1. The environmental system

Normal air in the troposphere contains 21% oxygen and 78% nitrogen (Altman and Dittman, 1966). As the concentration of oxygen decreases below 16% anoxia develops which affects body functions and brain centres (Patty, 1963). Life cannot be sustained when the oxygen concentration is below 6%, and immediate loss f consciousness results from exposure to a zero oxygen atmosphere. Air may also be the means for dispersal of toxic gases and particulates, microorganisms, and allergens.

Air has been considered an unlimited resource, but experience has shown the natural dispersion and cleaning machinists can be overtaxed in extensive localized areas. As the population multiplied and man's activities pollute the air in increasing quantities, there is potential danger of overloading the earth's atmosphere. Survival in individual cases without water may be measured in terms of days (depending on other factors); however, civilization cannot develop or prosper without ample water for domestic, agriculture, and commercial activities.

Many would specify recreational uses as a necessity. As with air, water may be the medium for transporting micro organisms and toxic chemicals. In many areas the quantity of water available is a serious problem, but in others water resources have been degraded beyond use by pollution resulting from man's activities. The attainment of an ample and proper diet is a serious health problem in many places throughout the world. Even the United States with its abundant food surpluses has found that in segments of its population 20-60% of the families had diets that fell short of providing the minimum requirements for adequate nutrition. No state is free from hunger. Expanding populations threaten to convert some of the best agricultural lands into sub divisions and industrial parks, which could have long-range implications for the food supply. Foods may be the mechanical means for conveying microorganisms and toxic substances.

Certain foods are also, under some circumstances, the media on which bacterial growth is sustained, with a resulting production of toxins. In many, if not most, areas of the world, shelter is necessary for man's survival. Shelter provides protection from excessive cold and heat, from the ravage of storms, and from environmental hazards. Properly designed shelter provides the spaces, services, safety, and privacy necessary for large numbers of people to live in close proximity to one another and in locations that would otherwise be uninhabitable. Broadly interpreted, shelter may be considered to include the house, the work place, recreational and transportation facilities, the space capsule, and the like.

Residues and Wastes

As man engages in the activities associated with living, wastes are produces. these are products which have no apparent useful purpose, or they are of such marginal utility that recovery is uneconomical. Such products include human, residential, agricultural, commercial and industrial wastes of all kinds. the continuous removal and safe disposal of these wastes is essential to the continued existence of any community may be overwhelmed and its citizens endangered. These wastes may be solid, liquid or gaseous.

Bodily discharges have historically been considered to be very hazardous to mankind. Intestinal diseases are readily transmitted where water or food is contaminated directed or indirectly by human wastes. Such wastes also provide a medium for fly breeding. Food scraps and waste food constitute garbage. When combined with other household waste, residential refuse is generated. The organic portion will attract and sustain flies and rats.

Where wastes are water-carried, pollution of water supplies may occur. Commercial and industrial liquid wastes may contain particulate and chemical pollutants. Many activities of man—driving an automobile, generating electric power, processing chemicals and petroleum, manufacturing certain products, disposal of wastes - may result, if uncontrolled, in the discharge of solid particles and gaseous pollutants to the atmosphere. Excessive pollution of the air has been cited as a cause of disease and death.

In summary, these wastes, if improperly handled endanger man's life support systems.

Environmental Hazards

Aside from deficiencies in the life support system, man is subjected to a variety of environmental hazards. Some of these are natural, but increasingly environmental hazards result from man's activities and numbers. Sometimes man-made hazards are direct in their impact on other men; but they may be indirect in their influence, acting through other biological systems or overburdening the capacity of natural systems for renewal, dispersion, or assimilation. The following factors can be used in categorizing environmental hazards: (1) biological; (2) chemical; (3) physical; (4) psychological; and (5) sociological.

Biological hazards are concerned primarily with the entry of disease producing infectious agents into man's body. Communicable diseases may be transmitted directly from one person to another by direct contact or aerosls discharged by sneezing or otherwise. Some times body discharges contaminate food or water consumed by the next victim or infect some other article with which the person has intimate contact. Where the environment may be modified to break the route of transmission from one person to another, such diseases may be prevented. Animal may be susceptible or the carriers of diseases (zoonoses) which may be transmitted to other animals and some of these diseases may be transmitted to man in a manner similar to the transmission of communicable diseases from man to man.

Diseases are also transmitted from person to person or from animals to man by means of other biological agents. In such cases, these agents are disease vectors. Among such diseases vectors are flies, which may mechanical, when they puncture the skin for a blood meal and later infect the victim in a similar manner. In the case of the mosquito, however, part of the life cycle of the disease-producing organisms (as in malaria) may take place in the mosquito before another person may be infected. Other common disease vectors include fleas, ticks,mites, cockroaches, etc.

Man is susceptible to invasion by worms which may produce dehabilitation or produce symptoms of disease. Such entry occurs through the ingestion of the eggs of the worms, or through penetration of the skin by the worms. Certain diseases are characterized by skin lesions and pustules. Organisms contained in these lesions may be deposited in ruptures of the skin of other persons or on vulnerable mucous membranes by direct intimate contact. Examples of such infections are syphilis and staphylococcus infections.

Host Source	*Modes of Transmission*	*Means of Entry*	*Receptor*
Man	Direct contact	Skin lesions	Man
or	Aerosols	Nose or Mouth	
Animal	Waters	Food or Water	
Arthropods	Skin puncture		

Fig. 2 Modes of transmission of communicable diseases.

There are other diseases which generally involve close person-to-person contact. Among these are infections of the upper respiratory tract, such as pneumoia, tuberculosis, and common colds, Aerosols composed of droplets discharged upon coughing, sneezing and breathing convey the organisms from one person to another. This transmission may be organisms from one person to another. This transmission may be aided by the use of common articles, such as drinking glasses, or by the contamination of foods.

Ordinarily, bacteria require moisture, a food medium, and proper temperature and pH to survive any length of time. Drying tends to kill the bacteria.

Communicable diseases are transmitted by the use of contaminated water for drinking, ablution and the preparation of food. Water supplies become contamined by receiving body discharges of man and animals. Bacteria are normally filtered out of water as it percolates through soils; however, water which follows passageways dissolved in limestone or fissures in rock formations will not be filtered.

Formations composed entirely of coarse gravels will also pass bacteria. Since many of the water-borne illnesses are of human rather than animal origin, the improper disposal of human wastes is the chief cause of contamination of the water. This may be from surface washings draining to a surface stream or entering underground supplies in limestone formations through sink holes. Shallow wells may become contaminated because the distance travelled through the soil is insufficient to filter out the bacteria. Wells which would otherwise produce safe water, by the use of contaminated water to prime pumps, or by contamination of ropes or buckets by unclean hands. Safe treated water may be contaminated through open reservoirs and by cross connections between the water pipes and waste piping. In the absence of organic matter to serve as food for the bacteria, there is a tendency for bacteria to die away in water.

Water-borne illnesses include hyphoid and paratyphoid fevers, cholera, bacillary dysentery, amoebic dysentery, and infectious hepatitis. The microorganisms causing these diseases are found in the intestinal and urinary discharges of infected persons. Some times persons may be carriers of these symptoms of the disease. Some of the communicable diseases generally transmitted by other means may be transmitted by water, e.g., undulant fever (brucellosis) and tularemia. Poliomyelitis is suspected of being capable of transmission by water.

Swimming or wading in water may provide the contact for the entry of certain helminths, e.g., dracotiaosis (Guinea worm disease), echinococcosis, and scistosomiasis. The helminths are usually encountered in the trophis, but scistosomiasis has been a problem in some waters of the United States. Food may be the means for the spread of infectious diseases in several ways. Consumption of the flesh of the infected animals, fowl, fish, or shellfish may result in the onset of a disease.

Food may simply become contaminated by spraying with aerosols produced by coughing, by handling with hands or equipment contaminated with disease organisms, or by incorporating contaminated water with the food. In some cases, food acts as a medium for the growth of disease organisms, producing large numbers of bacteria or toxins. Foodborne infections include such diseases as diphtheria and tuberculosis, as well as the intestinal diseases like typhoid fever and salmoculosis, dysentery undulant fever, Q fever, infectious hepatitis, leptospirosis, and botulism.

A storage or holding period after contamination of the food during which the bacteria multiply is not required in these cases, although some of the foodborne infections mentioned result from illness in the animal, e.g., the contamination of milk as a result of bovine tuberculosis or undulant fever in cattle. Salmonella may increase in such numbers after contamination of the food that gastrointestinal symptoms appear following ingestion. This is a food infection. Such foodborne infections are sometimes referred to as *food poisoning*, although this is not entirely correct. Strictly speaking, bacteria-caused food poisoning results from the growth of the bacteria in the food over a period of time during which the bacteria manufacture a toxin. When the food is ingested, food poisoning or intoxication results. Organisms frequently implicated are dstaphylococci and

Clostridium perfringens (welchii). *Under anaerobic conditions,* Clostridiu, boutlinum *produces a fatal toxin which is not heat stable.* Parasitic infections may be transmitted by foods which have contaminated. Diseased animals may be source of such infections if the meat is not thoroughly cooked, e.g., tapeworm and trichinosis.

some diseases may be transmitted through public water supplies, milk supplies, or other food. Characteristically, water-borne epidemics affect families on the distribution system, or in the system contaminated. Similarly, milkborne disease out-breaks tend to follow the milk routes, with additional cases where purchases are made at grocery stores or restaurants. Outbreaks due to the consumption of other foods will be scattered depending upon the residence of patrons of restaurants, guests at private diners, attendees at picnics, and patrons of certain stores, according to the food distribution system and the point at which contamination occurs. Preliminary judgments may be made by mapping the residence of cases.

Finding may be confirmed by taking case histories to identify common contacts and by bacteriological analyses of the water, milk and other food suspected. In recent years, the filtration and chlorination of water supplies and the pasteurization of milk have virtually eliminated water and milk as means for transmission of disease. Where disease outbreaks occur from water or milk customarily treated or pasteurized, there is usually a human or mechanical failure resulting in inadequate or no treatment, or there is gross contamination following the treatment process. Such sporadic outbreaks indicate the need for constant vigilance for the safety of water and milk supplies. In contrast to recent experience with water and milk, food poisoning outbreaks continue at an undesirable level.

There are a number of diseases of animals (zoonoses) which may be transmitted to man. This may be direct attack where the infectious agent is implanted in the wound. Rabies, rat-bite fever, and cat scratch fever fall into this category. Rabies, commonly associated with dogs, has been a hazards from bats and foxes and could involve other animals. As indicated in the discussion of food, man contracts some animal, as with brucellosis, Q fever, bovine tuberculosis, various tapeworms (beef, pork, fish), and salmonellosis.

Other animal diseases may be transmitted by direct contact, such as orthinosis (parrot fever or psittacosis), and by abrasions becoming infected, as anthrax (through skinning rabbits, etc.). Some diseases are conveyed from animals to man by anthropoids. These will be discussed under vector borne disease. It will suffice here to identify in this category the encephalitides, plague, murine typhus fever. Rocky Mountain spotted fever, relapsing fever, and tularemia. Obviously, some of the above diseases may be transmitted by more than one of the methods mentioned and sometimes by contact with waste discharges or food and water contaminated by such wastes.

Vector-borne diseases constitute threats throughout the world. While any animals may be considered disease vectors, this discussion is aimed at diseases carried by arthropods. With rapid transportation by airplane, arthropods may be carried everywhere unless strict precautions are taken. While much progress has been made in the United States in controlling such diseases as malaria, murine typhus fever, yellow fever, and bubonic plague, conditions exist which wound foster transmission if persons from other parts of the world, ill with any of these diseases, enter the community. Other vector-borne diseases do persis, such as the encephalitides, tularemia, and Rocky Mountain spoter fever. Plague exists in wild rodents in the sylvatic form in western states. Arthropods transmit diseases from animal to animal and from animal to man. By far the most important is the injection of the microorganisms in a wound made through the skin in the process of obtaining a blood meal. The mosquito is involved in this fashion in the transmission of malaria, yellow fever, dengue, filariasis, and he encephalitides, and similarly the rat flea in plague. Other diseases are transmitted by fleas, mites, and tics where organisms in feces deposited on the skin after a blood meal or from crushed body parts are rubbed into or otherwise gain entrance to the wound.

Epidemic typhus, murine typhus, scrub typhus, relapsing fever, Rocky Mountain spotted fever, and tularemia may be transmitted in this way. Arthropods may also be involved in the transmission of disease by simply transporting the organism from a source of infection (deposits of urine and feces) to hands, mouth, foods, or articles with which these come in contact. Such is the way that flied and roaches are involved in the spread of intestinal diseases-shigella dysentery, for example.

Contaminated soils offer the possibility of infection. Walking baefoot or lying on contaminated ground may provide the opportunity for entry of hookworm through the skin. Wounds and abrasions may be contaminated in the way, as well as others, with tentanus. Some persons are more seriously affected by communicable diseases than other. This may be related to their general state of health, concurrent diseases, physical vitality, natural or acquired immunity, possibly inherited factors, diet, environmental conditions, and other factors prevailing at the time of exposure. Thi is why some persons will become carriers, but not show symptoms of the disease; other will be ill to varying degrees; and still others die as a result. For many communicable diseases, immunizations have been developed which are highly effective in preventing illness completely or at least in minimizing the severity of the disease. However, besides being costly, it is difficult to maintain immunization in the total population.

Modern advances in medicine have resulted in a wide range of bactericidal therapeutic agents which are effective in abating disease in many instances. Unfortunately, some strains of the microorganisms develop resistance to these biological, rendering them ineffective, and in some instances persons develop allergies to certain biological when they have heavy or repeated doses. Thus the time has not yet arrived when we can depend solely upon immunization or therapeutics to solve the problem of communicable disease.

Where possible these measures should be supplemented by the maintenance of an environment in which communicable disease cannot persis or be transmitted. There are other biological hazards in the environment besides communicable diseases. There are the creatures whose venom is poisonous, e.g., certain snake,s scorpions, black widow spiders, and bees. Various plants berries, nuts and roots, such as horse chestnuts, toadstools and cator beans are poisonous to man.

Individuals may be allergic or acquire an allergy to many foods (eggs, wheat, etc.) to pollens of various plants (ragweed, roses, grasses, trees, etc.), to oils of plants (poison ivy, poison sumac and poison oak), to hair of dogs and cats, house dusts, the bite of insects and other arthropods, and the like. These allergies may manifest themselves by skin eruptions (hives), swelling or other symptoms (similar to respiratory or intestinal diseases).

While not directly related to disease of man, one may want to include in the consideration of biological environmental hazards the economic pests and insects. Pesticides are used to help control unwanted plants, animals and arthropods; however, unexpected and undesirable experiences in effects on wildlife have resulted from the indiscriminate use of pesticies. Research is being directed toward the development and use of natural biological control systems to avoid the problems resulting from chemical agents.

Excessive algal growths have been responsible for fishkills and bad tastes in water. The nuisance of mosquito bites has led to demands for control even where no mosquito borne disease is prevalent. Rats destroy valuable food and present a hazard of rat bites to infants, even when there is norat-borne disease. Perhaps man should be included in the biological hazards to man. With the decrease in other environmental hazards, some see man's continued high rate of reproduction as a serious threat. In some areas of the world, the increase in population has wiped out the benefits that might have been realized from economic development and the increase in food production.

The rate of increase in the numbers of people on earth began about 200 or 250 years ago to rise above earlier long-term averages. This rage of growth increased even more during the first half of this century and still more after World War II. Some authorities think this rate of growth (1.8% annual average 1950-1965) is nearing its climax. Estimates based on a 1.25% average annual increase forecast a range of about 4.4-7 billion for the year 2000.

The population of the world took more than a thousand years to double in the ages prior to 1750. Since then the population approximately doubled in the 150 years to 1900 and again in the years since then. Because of man's destructive habits with respect to other animals and plants,even fellow men, many are concerned about this upsetting of the balance of nature.

Chemical hazards are not new to mankind. Even before the rise of industry some waters were recognized as "bad." The term "miner's consumption" was a recognition that some activities held special peril even before the specific cause was unknown. Man's reaction to a chemical depends upon its toxicity and the individual's susceptibility, the duration of exposure, and the concentration of the chemical. The effect may be related to body weight and the form (solid, liquid, gas) of the chemical at the time of exposure. Occasionally, a slight tolerance may be developed over a period of time from small exposures, e.g. arsenic.

Some chemicals are more toxic when the subject is exposed to another chemical simultaneously (synergism). There are hundreds of new chemicals developed each year. For many of these, the toxicity may not be known in the development stages of production, with resulting occupational hazards. Many chemicals in liquid waste effluents find their way to water supplies; chemicals from industrial and auto exhausts are breathed; residues from agricultural pesticides are consumed with food. Even if there should prove to be no demonstrable harm from small increments in each of these elements water, air, food-who can say what the total effect may be over a number of years?

Natural exposures to toxic chemicals may occur where water dissolves the chemical in percolating through the ground. High concentrations of nitrates (methemo-globinemia-"blue babies") and fluoride (mottled tooth enamel) may be acquired in this way. Volcanoes are about the only natural source of toxic gases, unless one considers the gases freed in the mining of coal (mainly methane). Among the toxic substances encountered through breathing are chemically active dust (e.g. lead), gases (e.g., chlorine, carbon monoxide), solvent vapors (mainly hydrocarbons and chlorinated hydrocarbons). Some chemical substances may be absorbed through the skin, particularly solvents. Where gases or solvent vapors are heavier than air, in addition to any possible toxicity their presence may displace all of the oxygen.

Displacement may also occur in sewers, as methane gas is produced in the biological decomposition of the sewage, and sometimes in the cleaning of large tanks or vessels, where vapors of the chemical stored or of the solvent used for cleaning fill the space. If a person enters an atmosphere with zero oxygen, he immediately loses consciousness. A gas mask does not help a rescuer since he requires an air supply. Some gases are irritating at low concentrations,but at higher concentrations hydrogen sulfide may be fatal, and nitrogen dioxide may cause ensilage disease among workers in silos. Allergic reactions may occur after chemical contact depending on individual sensitivity.

Chemicals may concentrate in certain issues of plants, animals and fish. As higher forms of life consume lower forms, and the big eat the little, successive concentrations may result in a tenfold increase over the initial concentration. Thus, pesticides washing into a stream may not result in a high concentration at that point, but, through biological concentration, fish or shellfish may become hazardous to man or other life.

Chemicals discharged to the atmosphere may undergo reactions in the presence of moisture or when irradiated by sunlight. Polluted reducing atmospheres, of the New York and London type, have been held responsible for high rates of emphysema and bronchial diseases. The primary pollutants are particulate matter and oxides of sulfur. These occurrences are not well understood at present since the laboratory experiments conducted have failed to reproduce the ill effects of polluted community air at comparable concentrations.

An association between the occurrence of lung cancer and cigarette smoking has been observed, but it has also been noted that urban inhabitants have lung cancer more frequently than rural residents. Some authorities suggest this "urban factor" may be the result of air pollution. Although some chemicals may be hazardous, the proper use of some of these same chemicals can enhance the quality of life. Nitrogen in fertilizer is necessary to the production of crops, but an over-abundance,while increasing the crops yield, will also result in a build-up of nitrates in the ground water.

Chlorine is used to destroy pathogens in drinking water and swimming pools and to oxidize wastes but when inhaled is extremely toxic. Too much fluoride in a natural wastes will mottle tooth enable; but when the fluoride content is adjusted to the proper range, tooth decay is prevented and no mottling occurs. While food additives are sometimes questionable, many are beneficial in lengthening shelf life (preservatives) or improving the nutritive qualities (vitamin additions).

Physical hazards in the environment may cause death, disease, or disability. These concerns include a wide range of factors such as dusts, humidity, equipment and environmental design, and radiation. In the previous paragraphs, chemically active dusts were considered. There are other dusts which are not absorbed in the body but cause a fibrosis when deposited in the lungs-silica, asbestos, etc. Some dusts, e.g., cement dust, however, may be a nuisance, but, a far as we know, do not induce a disease.

Temperature and humidity are important to efficient human performance. The critical air temperature for man ranges from 1°C to 32°C and the thermoneutrality zone is 24°-31°C. Metabolic rate, oxygen consumption, respiration, heart beat, and blood pressure are affected by temperature. Temperature cooling control is not usually specified in housing regulations, although excessive numbers of persons die in summer heat wave. Length of exposure to extremes of temperature and humidity is critical.

Electromagnetic radiation includes X-rays, ultraviolet, infrared, and microwaves. Prolonged exposure may induce skin burns, cause elevation in temperature and even death, X-rays cause effects similar to Y-rays as both are ionizing radiations. Carefully controlled ionizing radiation is invaluable in making radiographic pictures and in therapy; however, excessive exposures may induce cancers, cause genetic mutations and other biological damage.

Mechanical vibration and noise can cause hearing loss and produce other psychological and physical disturbances. People living in cities may suffer some hearing loss from community noise. The physical design of the equipment and environment may effect the probability of accidents.

Machinery, automobiles, highways, homes, and recreational facilities should be designed to prevent the occurrence of accidents. Accidents are the leading cause of death in most age groups, particularly young adults. Inspite of this fact, only recently has accident control been considered a public health concern. Light, colour, contrast and glare are important in visual tasks from the standpoint of efficiency, fatigue, perception, and comfort. 'Biological systems are sensitive to changes in atmospheric pressure. Furthermore, a rapid decrease of air pressure may result in the release of nitrogen bubbles in the blood stream causing "bends." It is generally conceded that exercise is essential to the maintenance of a status of health and in the prevention or delay of some degenerative diseases of the middle and later years of life. Thus, the availability of recreational opportunities and facilities that allow for physical exercise is important, particularly in the urban environment.

Sociological and Psychological parameters of environmental design are not as well delineated as biological, chemical and physical factors. A total consideration of the environment of man must consider sociological and Psychological influences (and hazards), even though we may not at this time know their precise effect, the magnitude of their influence, or the epidemiology of mental illness. There is enough information available to suggest that this is an area of serious concern. Dubos asserts that mental characteristics are shaped by the environment, that genes only determine responses to stimuli. Envrionmental stimuli impinge on man from the time of conception. On the other hand, a variety of environmental stimuli are necessary for mental development.

Even though man may adapt to Envrionmental conditions this does not occur without stresses which may ultimately result in disorders of the body and mind. Studies on this subject are difficult to evaluate because of the multiplicity of variables that cannot be isolated to study specific effects. One study found that four out of five inhabitants of a highly congested area had psychiatric disorders, with one in four sufficiently severe to disrupt their daily lives, compared to a low density agrarian community where 97% never experienced a major mental disorder. Noise, overcrowding, lack of privacy, lack of opportunity for social interaction, lack of open space, boredom, compulsory leisure, tedium in travelling from home to work, stresses from work, traffic, crowds, and "estrangement from the conditions and natural cycles under which human evolution took place" are environmental factors which have been identified as having possible social and psychological consequences. Determination of the sociological and psychological parameters of environmental design will require more definitive research. Findings from studies with animals and some studies of human population indicate that sociological and psychological hazards are just as important as the biological, chemical, and physical factors in the development of positive health and in the prevention disease.

A primary objective of environmental control is to prevent disease. This means that man must be prevented from encountering the hazards or the hazard must be removed from the community. Of course, it is preferable to percent an environmental condition even arising which is hazardous to man. While prevention of hazardous conditions is essential, this is only half the job. It should be a public policy to provide an environment which maximizes man's health. A desirable environment should provide a variety of compatible stimuli that are necessary to mental and physical development. It must also provide for the fundamental physiological needs of man. Environmental hazards vary in their manifestation, but one or more of certain fundamental principles of environmental control are generally applicable. These include (1) isolation; (2) substitution; (3) shielding (4) treatment; and (5) prevention.

Isolation protected man from epidemics before the rise of cities and the mobility of populations. However, populations which developed under isolated conditions were extremely vulnerable to the ravages of disease when it was introduced to the community. Natural waters remote from human habitation may be safe to drink because no source of disease organisms exists. Populations remote from mosquito breeding area are not subject to mosquito-borne diseases. Under present conditions, isolation (separation by distance) is not generally reliable means of environmental protection, although there are some exceptions where isolation may be useful. In some areas, watersheds are fenced in and people excluded. Such policies are often criticized, however,because some people want to use reservoirs for recreation, such as boating, fishing, and swimming. In protecting against ionizing radiation, heated surfaces, and other conditions where effects diminish with distance, isolation is a useful procedure.

A variety of hazardous operations may be conducted in an isolated location such that the general population is not exposed to the hazard. (Other precautions must be taken for the protection of those in the hazardous area). Military personnel who are disciplined may be ordered not to go into mosquito-infested areas, but restriction of movement is not usually applicable to civilian populations. There has been circumstances where public swimming at polluted beaches and in polluted streams and lakes has been prohibited. Such orders are difficult to enforce.

Substitution is frequently a low cost, easily applied, completely effective method of environmental control. A simple application is the substitution of a harmless cleaning fluid for a toxic one. The use of food which do not support the rapid growth of staphylococcus organisms may be effective in the prevention of food poisoning. On a broader scale, a non polluted water supply may be developed in preference to a polluted one, and a chemical manufacturing process may be substituted for one that creates air, water or land pollution. The substitution of degradable detergents for nondegradable ones is a case in point.

Shielding, as used here, is distinct from isolation. Shielding is the use of barriers for protection while a person remains in relatively close proximity to the hazard. Safety glasses and protective clothing are personnel measures which may be employed. Screening for the exclusion of mosquitoes and flies and heat shields are other examples. On cafeteria lines glass sneeze guard are used to protect against food contamination. Lead is used to restrict the emission of stray ionizing radiation from X-ray machines.

Where other measures are not applicable, treatment of the hazard may employed. Environmental treatment methods,which may be used in conjunction with dilution or dispersion of contaminating substances or prophylaxis, include: (1) destruction; (2) conversion; (3) removal; and (4) inhibition. Complete destruction is applicable particularly to biological hazards. Boiling and cooking employ heat to kill microorganisms.

Autoclaving employs heat and pressure. Pasteurization employs sufficient heat to kill pathogenic or other undesirable microorganisms, but necessarily all organisms. Microorganisms may also be killed by oxidation using chlorine or a similar substance. Other chemicals are sued as disinfectants, algacides, fungicides, bactericides, pesticides, larvicides, rodenticides, etc. Certain animal diseases, such as bovine tuberculosis and undulant fever, are controlled by periodic testing and killing of infected animals. Eradication is sometimes attempted for weeds, mosquitoes, and rats.

Conversion of harmful substances to less harmful or harmless substances usually involves chemical or biochemical processes. Strongly acid and strongly alkaline liquid wastes may be mixed together in a way to neutralize each other. On other circumstances, various methods of chemical treatment may be employed to induce a desired reaction and conversion. Where substances are biodegradable the conversion may be accomplished by the use of microorganisms.

Odorous organic air pollutants may be oxidized by combustion at high temperature or with a catalyst at lower temperatures. Removal of harmful substances from water and air may be accomplished by a variety of methods. Sedimentation and filtration result inthe removal of solid particles. Chemicals may cause coagulation and precipitation for removal of soluble substances and as aids to sedimentation. In exchange is used in water treatment, and electrostatic precipitation in air cleaning. Bag filters and cyclones are used for mechanical separation of particles in air streams. Scrubbers may be used for mechanical and chemical treatment of air streams.

While removal of harmful substances from water and air streams may prevent air and water pollution, there is usually a residue remaining for some ultimate disposal. Deposition of waste products on land may create other hazards which restricts the use of this method of disposal to isolated areas. Population increases augment the waste disposal problems to such a degree that there is now intense pressure to recycle waste products and use them as raw materials. Consequently, simple removal is not an ultimate solution to many environmental problems, but it must be coupled with a conversion process to produce something useful, or at least, harmless.

Inhibition may be used where an environmental threat exists, but its effects may not materialize or may be minimized by environmental intervention. Thus pH controls or the addition of salt or sugar may be used in food preservation. If bacteria contaminate the food, they are unlikely to persist in the unfavourable environment created. Refrigeration, while not destructive of bacteria, may inhibit the growth of bacteria and the production of toxins. The foregoing treatment methods are used to eliminate or reduce the gross quantity of the contaminate in the environment. To a degree any alternative approach which resulted in a lower level of concentration of a contaminate in the environment might have a comparable effect. For example, if the discharge of a liquid waste was proportioned according to stream flow, the resultant concentration in the stream might not be harmful.

To regulate the discharge of the waste may require storage facilities so that the discharge could be with held during periods of low stream flow. Air contaminate storage is not feasible, but conceivably operations could be shut down or curtailed during periods of stagnant air with similar effects. This approach uses dispersion or dilution to minimize the effects of environmental pollution by maintaining a relatively low concentration of pollution. There is much philosophical controversy about this approach. There are advocates of the use of the "natural assimilative capacity' of the environment. Directly opposed are the advocates of a "no degradation" policy.

Quite different from dispersion is the use of masking agents. The massing agents do nothing to reduce the level of the contaminate. They only inhibit the sensory perception of the presence of the pollutant. As such, they could be hazardous. Masking agents are used frequently to hide unpleasant odours. It would be better to eliminate the odour source and to improve ventilation for interior spaces.

Minimizing exposure through restriction of activities immunization against disease and the use of prophylactic agents may avoid infections and, so such, are measures which may be used to avoid the effects of environmental hazards. One may use only boiled water and cooked food when travelling in areas where drinking water is not safe or sewage is used to irrigate low growing vegetables. The avoidance of unpasteurized milk and uncooked shellfish are similar practices. Restraints of this type are unacceptable to many people. Immunizations are available for many communicable diseases transmitted through the environment.

If immunization is developed before entering an area where a disease is endemic, one will not likely develop the disease and, if one does, the severity may be minimized. Immunization is used also to control disease while environmental control measures are being instituted and where environmental control measures fail. Where immunization is not available, prophylactic agents may be used to avoid becoming ill with the disease. This is practiced to protect military personnel going into areas where malaria is endemic.

2 ENVIRONMENTAL HEALTH PROBLEMS IN INDIA

The situation in our country is indeed unique in as much as we are developing among deveioped world but developed inthe developing world. It is a country where centuries co-exist and we have today both near-stone age to near-space age cultures. Obviously, the spectrum of diseases ranges from those that result from poverty and stark need, to those that are the result of prosperity, affluence and greed. Clearly, the challenges faced by our medical scientists and health planners are considerable. The state of health of the people does not depend only on the number of doctors and hospitals, but also on clean environment because if it is conducive to spread of disease, the state of health of the people will be poor.

The system has to be preventive as also curative and both are important. Nearly 80 per cent of world's diseases more so in developing world, can be linked with water. In our country, there are 14 river systems which account for 83 per cent of land mass, 80 per cent of population and 85 percent of water discharge. A detailed analysis, based on our monitoring status, shows that 90 per cent of pollution load in river system is on account of human waste, to be precise, faecal matter. In this regard out biggest defaulters are the City Municipalities. Clean drinking water and sanitation therefore, get equal emphasis as number of hospitals and doctors. In fact, doctors can do precious little if there is a constant source of infection.

A simple illustration is 'Kumbh' when coliform increases from 300/100 ml to about 165,000/100 ml. The infection persists for 335-50 kms downstream. Here then is a situation where infection is in a concentrated form. Infant mortality is of the order of 125/100. Consider the perception of a villager in this regard. His requirement is for at least five children. One each for firewood collection, tending cattle work in the field, domestic chores and for general (market purposes). He needs 2-3 more as a buffer or standby on account of high child mortality. His view is that five children provide him with only five children provide him with only five mouths but ten working hands. There is another facet of this problem as seen from the following tabulation:

	National average	UP	Kerala
Death rate			
1981-83	14.4	15.7	6.6
Birth rate			
1981	35.9	40.4	28.1
Infant mortality			
1981	126	160	37

A perusal of the above table shows that Kerala has significantly lower rates than even the national average. The reasons are high rate of literacy in women, better environmental sanitation and Government assured food supply. Even in Punjab, figures are higher than Kerala though Punjab is the grannery of Indian with a very high rate of economic development. Social status and education of women is indeed a vital factor. However, we tend to ignore the role women have in our social, cultural and economic milieu. The lesson we draw is that health/medicare cannot be looked at in isolation, and we need to blame doctors if socio-economic and sanitary conditions are poor in villages. Again, the different types of diarrheas, which by themselves may not be killers, could prove disastrous when accompanied by malnutrition, and 15 lakh children die of this in the pre-school group i.e, about three children per minute. Since we do not take a holistic view, diarrhea is almost a permanent epidemic.

A similar situation is seen regarding the Guinea Worm. Nearly 8000 villages in Rajasthan and Central India are afflicted with the disease. Infection although water containing cyclops which feeds on larvae of this form. Prevention of disease is well within comprehension and competence and is neither difficult nor expensive. It is essentially a questions of supply of clean water accompanied by sanitation. In this connection, it may be pointed out that the condition of the water pipes in major cities is far from satisfactory.

There is correlation between intermittent water supply and hepatitis. When there is no weather in the pipes, due to reverse pressure the empty pipes draw subsoil water full of sewage and faecal matter. This is the source of infection. Thus, there is a serious gap between proper water supply and sewerage system, and usually water is provided to the exclusion of sewerage facility. A report from WHO shows a direct association between distance of water supply and the extent of diarrhoea ie, incidence is minimum if the tap is nearby, but maximum if far away. besides, the question of personal hygiene also figures.

There is yet another aspect of environmental health: that malaria has returned and filaria and Japanese encephalitis and Kalaazar are all increasing. Malignant malaria or chloroquine-resistant malaria is around Delhi.

Contrary to the views of Sharma and Mehrotra, there is a general belief that there is a correlation between the spread of these diseases and spread of irrigation and pesticide. If true, these are the negative impacts of agriculturisation. Here then is a dilemma.

On the one hand, we are critically balanced in agricultural production vis-a-vis our population explosion. On the other hand, land resource is finite and production per unit time and land must go up. This meas enhanced use of agricultural chemicals (pesticides and fertilizers) as also water. This indicates chances of increased pesticide resistance, water logging and high salinization. These situations are conductive to the spread of water-borne diseases. A recent case of this nature is seen in Malnad. Here, rich paddy farmers have taken to high yielding rice culture with high inputs of chemicals. The rich farmers have stopped giving food for wages to the labourers, who began eating crabs in the rice fields which had high DDT and BHC content.

The labour community, being highly inbred, are easily susceptible to disease. In most cases, pain began in hips and knees and soon the afflicted persons could not even stand up. This incident shows how vulnerable our poor are to socio-economic and environmental changes. What are the lessons we draw from the foregoing account ? Firstly, future impact assessment of all development projects must include health aspects as well. In fact, medical experts must be an integral component of all our environmental impact assessments. Secondly habitat management is very vital as this can lead to breeding grounds for mosquitoes and increased salination and water logging leads to formation of wet deserts. Thirdly, disease control cannot be taken up successfully in isolation. this has to be a corporate effort. To doctors, health educators, social anthropologists, media men, engineers, socioeconomic and other. It also involves habitat change and population migration, water supply, sanitation, human settlements, socio-economic conditions and the level of education particularly of women. Frothily, health care is biased towards the cities rather than villages as there are nearly 5,100 hospitals for 109 million urban people whereas only 5,400 health centres for 439 million rural people.

In sum and substance, the root cause is the demographic pressure. Imagine the situation if we were half as many people in India today. Our problems would have been considerably less. Here then is an areas which can be ignored only at our peril. Many revolutionary researches are on the anvil in the area of bio-technology which may help in population control. Thus we can list six conclusions regarding the state of environmental health of India:

(a) "India faces a disastrous `double burden' of disease. Most of the old diseases continue to be rampant,while new ones are making rapid strides. The Indian death rate is no longer going down.

(b) Every third persons who dies in India is a child below the age of five; a victim of a vicious combination of poverty malnutrition insanitary environment and unclean drinking water.

(c) Diarrhoeas attack children in particular. Three die every minute, about 1.5 million every year. This constitutes a permanent epidemic in our country.

(d) The extension of irrigation in creating excellent breeding grounds for disease carriers, including the mosquitoes that spread the fatal disease Japanese encephalitis, almost unknown in India 30 years ago. Every third person in India now lives in danger of falling prey to filariasis.

(e) With water pipes empty most of the time and sewage seeping into them, hepatitis is increasing by leaps. This disease is not yet a notifiable disease.

(f) Increasing use of cigarettes and bidis and greater use of chemicals because of industrialisation already results in half a million deaths from cancer every year. By the end of the century, India could be an unenviable country with so called diseases of poverty and of affluence coexisting with each other".

The quality of life is directly related to the quality of the environment. Concepts of "pure" water, "pure" food, "clean" air, "clear" neighborhood reflect the newer concepts of health as meaning more than the absence of disease. the environment must satisfy not only man's physiological needs but also his psychological and sociological needs.

The quality of the environment through history has been a measure of the character of a civilization - "a way of life". Levels of concern for environmental quality heave been classified roughly as follows (1) bare survival-control of major epidemics of disease and violent death, minimum food and water, (2) control of disease and injury - control of endemic and dietary disease and accidental injury; (3) efficient performance-adequate and proper diet, maintenance of environment for efficient use of manpower; and (4) comfort-stimulating environment, aesthetic satisfactions, comfort control. The first of these-bare survival-is a rather precarious existence. Any failure results in premature death for many people. Although we pride ourselves on the achievements of our civilization, there are many places in the world where this first level of environmental quality has yet to be attained.

Too often solutions of problems on a piecemeal basis generate new environmental problems in other areas.

Consequently, it is necessary to take an ecological approach to environmental quality and consider the totality of the environment with man as part of an ecosystem. While geographical approaches have been characteristic of the past, in future years the population increase will require that the environment of the world be reviewed as closed system. Man has the capacity, but it remains for him to exercise his will and wisdom, to modify the environment for the maximization of his physical, mental, and social well-being.

3 Habitat

In a country like India, urban poverty and rural urban migration are closely related. When cities grow at yearly rates of 5 percent or more, as Bombay, Calcutta, Madras, Delhi, Hyderabad, Bangalore. Ahmedabad have over the last three decades, at least half the growth is caused by net 'in-migration', concentrated very heavily in prime working areas, swelling the urban labour force, holding down wages and incomes in the urban economy, staraining housing and related urban to their limit.

Growth in Population of Major Indian Cities ('000)

	1901	1951	1961	1971	1981	1991
Calcutta U.A.	1488	4589	5737	7081	9166	10860
Greater Bombay	813	2967	4152	5971	8203	12569
Delhi U.A.	214	1437	2359	3637	5752	8375
Madras U.A.	594	1542	1945	3170	4277	5361
Hyderabad U.A.	448	1128	1249	1796	2566	4273
Ahmedabad U.A.	186	877	1206	1742	2515	3279
Bangalore	159	779	1200	1654	2914	4108
Kanpur U.A.	203	705	971	1275	1685	2103
Pune U.A.	164	608	791	1135	1685	2444
Nagpur	128	449	644	930	1298	1657

But the belief that such migrants are unemployed parasites is absolutely incorrect. Survey results from Calcutta, Bombay, Delhi and Madras clearly show that most migrants find jobs fairly quickly, suggesting prearranged employment. A recent study of unemployment in calcutta, for instance found that unemployment was high among urban born educated youth but very low among the poorer sections. Muslim migrants from Bihar and eastern Uttar Pradesh were largely absorbed in the city's jute industry. Hindus from rural Bengal were concentrated in the engineering, chemicals, rubber and printing industries. Calcutta's rickshaw pullers are lagregly migrants from Bihar and Orissa.

The occupations of plumbers,domestic servants and paanwallas are dominated by people from Orissa, and tanning and leather works are largely a Bihar Muslim activity. Vast occupational networks are at work among the poor to find work for the newcomer. In Bombay, textile mill workers are mainly from the Maharashtra districts of Ratnagiri, Sangli and Satara. Construction workers are largely from Andhra Pradesh. Restaurant and catering industry jobs are cornered by young migrants from Udupi, Karanataka. Pannwallas and roadside food vendors are usually 'bhaiyas' from Uttar Pradesh.

A study of Bombay's labour market points out that less than 15 percent of the poor migrants studied were employed, and that most of them regarded themselves as better off for having moved to the city. This study shows that the duration for which a migrant remains unemployed is related to the resourcefulness and "influence of friends and relatives." Majority of the migrants (77.7 percent) have some support during the period of waiting (for a job). Family members and relatives from the largest single source which helped 45 percent of the migrants. Caste fellows and friends from the native place each halped 11 percent of the migrants get jobs. Of those with none to support them 61 percent took up employment (usually of the casual variety) immediately.

The cities, compared with the villages, promise lighter work and higher and steadier wages. A study from Delhi states that the migrants' average earnings over the year were two and a half times more than what they could earn in the rural area. Many or most migrants see urban earnings as supplementing the rural, their urban stay as temporary and their places of origin as their permanent homes. Thus, the migrants range from the seasonal or shuttle migrant coming for a few months to the permanent settler seeking a new way of life. Seasonal or short-term migration is usually resorted to by agricultural labourers, tenant farmers and small landholders during slack cultivation seasons.

Many rural workers rely partly on farming and partly on some trade, craft or service skill, and their nonagricultural occupations may take them periodically to neighbouring towns and cities. Then there are 'target migrants': those who come with a specific purpose in mind, usually to earn a lumpsum of money for marriages or agricultural investment, and plan to return home once that is achieved. Target migrants may sometimes stay in the city for several years. The most substantial section, however, are the "working life migrants", who move to the cities for the rest of their working lives. But they keep in close touch with their places of origin, often leave part of their nuclear families there, and plan to retire at home.

The bhaiyas of Uttar Pradesh, as they are called in Bombay, epitiomise the working life migrant. William Rowe has provided a very vivid portrait of the migrant bhaiya as seen from the vantage point of on Uttar

Pradesh village called Senapur : "It is recurrent rather that permanent' because these men traditionally go to the city without their wives and families and return home annually for visits of a month or six weeks.

With few exceptions these men view migration to the city as a temporary solution to economic problems and maintain their involvement in the network of personal relationships in the villages. In several cases they have worked for 25-30 years in Bombay which is 900 miles from the village... migrants to the city either remit or bring home with them all of their income beyond their minimum living expenses. This income has a differential function for the various families and caste communities who have deputed migrants to the city. Some men are pulled to the city because it is here that money can be earned to improve the family position at home (through purchase of additional land of farm animals or other capital expenditure)."

Given that kind of attitude of life, how do the slum dwellers themselves look at their unstable huts? The startling answer turn up by studies is that they do not really think it is such a terrible problem. The poor city bound migrants come from mud huts in the villages and expect little more, at least upon arrival. Village water supplies are neither more accessible nor much purer than those of the city. Lavatories and waste disposal systems are usually nonexistent back home.

A second factor is the correlation between caste religious status and housing quality. In Hyderabad, for instance, 59 percent of slum dwellers are estimated to be from the scheduled castes and tribes, and 34 percent are Muslims. In many parts of India, especially in the villages, prior to independence Harijans were forbidden to build solid dwellings. They were forced to live in huts and forbidden to use common village wells. In that context the Harijans in cities may not feel so deprived today as outside observers might imagine. The urban poor can therefore tolerate slum conditions better than the urban rich. On occasions, when government housing programmes have allowed other housing choices to slum dwellers, many of them have sold out their official houses and returned to their original slums.

Research and interviews with groups of squatters conducted by Meera Bapat in Pune's slum clearly indicated that their principal concern is employment, housing is second. They seek the crowded, inner-city locations because the chances of finding jobs, especially the unskilled, casual jobs for which they are most eligible are so much higher in the central business district than anywhere else. In a national survey of settlement patterns of the urban poor, Rakesh Mohan (housing expert and constant Planning Commission) has concisely summarised the underlying logic and evolving priorities. "To poorest (for example, fresh migrants) are mainly interested in location.

Being near job markets saves on transport costs. In their highly uncertain situation the only security they are inerested in is job security. Their meagre income only allows for food consumption and other bare essentials in a kind of lexicographic ordering. The only amenity they need is space for sleeping. The next group, with a reasonably stable income put still not well-off, is inerested in security of tenure. A temporary jobless does not then mean displacement of residence as well. They are also more interested in space than amenities and are willing to pay for it. Finally the richest, low income group is more interested in amenties, having a stable income and subsistence essentials. Electricity, plumbing, well-designed housing and receation then become important and will be demanded by this group."

Slum Population Growth in Some Major Indian Cities

Metropolitan City	Year	Polulation of City	Slum Populations (millions)	%of Slum Population (millions)
Calcutta	1974	3.19	1.44	45.00
	1981	9.16	3.24	35.35
Greater Bombay	1976	7.94	3.24	41.00
	1981	8.2	4.20	51.03
Delhi	1977	5.29	1.32	25.00
	1981	5.71	3.02	53.00
Madras	1977	2.47	0.99	40.09
	1981	4.27	1.36	31.86
Hyderabad	1977	1.99	0.4	20.00
	1981	1.51	0.66	25.16
Kanpur	1976	1.33	0.56	41.98
	1981	1.68	0.68	40.34

But central land is most likely to be owned either privately or by the government, squeezing the squatter out. The slum dweller sees the makeshift hut, often on encroached land, as a solution rather than a problem. It may be ugly, insanitary, illegal, but it does nevertheless serve as a shelter.

There are thus two major aspects of the housing crisis. On the one hand, the failure of the government to view urban housing as a multidimensional process which involves making provision for several other needs apart from physical shelter as a result, after 35 years of governmental planning. There is a colossal housing and infrastructural shortage which has steadily accumulated over the years and is now, as the Planning Commission itself admits, beyond solution. On the other hand, the urban poor have solved this problem in their own desperate manner, by building clusters of hutments and shanties wherever and however they can. The resulting slums, barring a South African type authoritarian 'solution', are here to stay. Give this grim scenario, Indian should perhaps learn to live with slums.

Planners are also beginning to realise that squatters are economically valuable citizens who add to the gross national product by constructing their own shelter, no matter how make-shift, which saves the government a considerable amount of money. That squatters are upwardly mobile citizens in search of economic oportunity and have demonstarted high levels of enterprise, tenacity, and ability to suffer acute hardships; that the informal sector in which a majority of the slum dwellers are economically active contributes significantly to the city's overall economic growth; and that they should be helped and not hindered. What can be done is to upgrade, not demolish, most existing slums, and move the remaining squatters and pavement dwellers to reasonably well-located vacant lands as part of a site-and-services scheme. In at least a few cities, local governments are attempting to act on these views and help the urban poor settle down.

Ahmedabad, Calcutta, Madras and Hyderabad are experimenting with slum upgrading programmes. There are two basic elements; security of tenure and improvement of the physical conditions and basic amenities. The experience of these cities merit attention both as examples of what is possible with all the constraints, and as alternative to the constraints, and as alternative to the essentially demolition and eviction-oriented policies of Bombay and Delhi.

The squatter relocation project in Vasna suburb

combines self-help with government assistance. With about 2.25 million people in the metropolitan region, Ahmedabad has about 7000 slums and sqatter settlements, housing nearly 415,000 people. After the 1973 floods in the city's Sabarmati river which washed away thousands of squatter homes, the Ahmedabad Study Action Group (ASAG), a voluntary interdisciplinary organisation of various professionals, submitted to the municipal authorities an integrated plan for moving the displaced squatters to a new suburban settlement. Their plan involved building for them new homes and providing social and economic welfare assistance to raise their living standards and their ability to participate in the city's economic activity.

A constant refrain of the ASAG proposals was that 'slums are people, not places'. The state government was eventually pushed into allocating 43 acres for a new settlement located about 7 km. from the city centre. The Ahmedabad municipality agreed to extend piped water, sewerage, street lighting, roads, and community facilities such as schools, shops and health centres. HUDCO (Housing and Urban Development Corporation) approved low iterest 20 years loans to the occupants which was followed by state subsidy of Rs. 700 per family and another Rs. 400 per family was provided by Oxfam. A majority of the flood dislocated squatters agreed to move to Vasna.

The results, nine years after the first bricks were laid in May 1974, have, however, been mixed. Problems of quality of shelter construction, distance from the city and employment sites, an artificial juxtaposition of diverse ethnic/cast groups,incomplete city drainage facilities, differing economic and social priorities among the squatters themselves, and political corruption have marred the project. Many of the original squatters have returned to locations closer to the city centre. Other people have moved in and the neighborhood now is ethnically more homogenous in Muslims now forming 75 percent of its residents. Despite these problems and changes, however, Vasna remains a very interesting experiment.

In 1971 the Calcutta Metropolitan Development Authority (CMDA) started the country's most ambitious slums upgrading programme to cover in stages, by 1984, the city's slum population of approximately three million. By 1980 the total slum population had risen to 2.7 million crammed into some 3,000 separate slums. Calcutta's planners have tried to improve the exiting slum environment and make it more livable.

The CMDA has focussed on six areas: conversion of existing service latrines to sanitary latrines and the construction of a new toilet for every 25 persons: potable water tap connection to individual huts or for every 100 persons with an average water supply of 90 litres per heads; surface drainge facilities through underground conducts connected to an underground sewer system wherever available, or open surface drain discharging into the nearest open drainage channels; paving of roads, streets and pathways; and miscellaneous facilities such as garbage vats, dustbins and batching facilities at suitable locations. These basic civic services cost Rs. 120 per person between 1971 and 1973, rising to Rs. 150 later.

As the programme spread away from areas with basic infrastructure, the cost rose to Rs. 350 as totally new facilities had to be installed. By 1981 some 1.9 million slum inhabitants had been serviced at a total cost of Rs. 25 crore. "Implementing the programme was a huge technological challenge", says M.S. Moitra, Director General (Operations) of the CMDA and the brain behind the project. For instance, as most slums were not served by the city systems, captive sewer systems had to be designed for entire slums, by which the slums sewage was collected by interconnecting pipes and then dumped into the nearest city sewer. Cheap latrines were bulk manufactured. Unfortunately, the problems remain: some 70 percent of the assets created are out of order at any given time. Thousands of latrines are choked with excreta and garbage. Taps stay dry.

Drains overflow after slight rain. Uncovered manholes are safety hazards. Street lights are without power, the blocked latrines and leaking sewer pipes have sometimes led to spate of cholera and diarrhoea in recent years. "It would cost only Rs. 3 per household per year to maintain these services," says Moitra. "The existing system of entrusting contractors with responsibility for maintaining services is inefficient and costly. "The CNDA has spent Rs. 25 crore on a Rs. 5 crore job. The rest of the money has simply been siphoned off on contracts." A World Bank mission even took note of this recently. Proposals to involve the community in maintenance have not been welcomed, in fear that the politicians would lose their clout.

In 1971, the Tamil Nadu Slum Clearance Board (TNSCB) decided to resettle all hutment slum dwellers of Madras city—about 0-74 million people at the time in pucca tenements to be constructed with public funds by 1977. By 1978, instead of the 1,64,000 tenements planned at an estimated cost of Rs. 164 crore, barely 23,000 were actually completed at a cost of Rs. 25 crore.

The authorities shifted their emphasis to upgradation from 1977 onwards, encouraged by a World Bank loan. The two major schemes are the Enviornmental Improvement Scheme (EIS) and the World Bank Improvement Scheme (WBIS). Under the EIS, 293 slums were covered to benefit about 1.05 lakh households at an estimated cost of Rs. 5.12 crore. The local authorities soon realised that the funds would not provide adequate services for all the beneficiary households. The amount spent varied considerably, less than Rs. 100 per household in some slums to Rs. 1,300 per household in others. The average expenditure was about Rs. 500 per household. A survey of the actual improvements in 23 slums was carried out in 1980 by the Operations Research Group (ORG), an independent research unit, which found that less than Rs. 625 per household had actually been spent in 90 percent of the slums.

The report contrasts the case of VOC Nagar where expenditure was the highest, Rs. 1,300 per household, with Karunanidhi Nagar, where it was Rs. 500 per household. While VOC Nagar's 490 households had been provided with baths and lavatories, stormwater drains, roads and wells, their less favoured counterparts in Karunanidhi Nagar were provided with only stormwater drains and roads. Maintenance has been neglected. The 1980 survey of VOC Nagar found "the baths, latrines and wells under disuse, the roads broken and full of ditches and stormwater drains in no condition to clear stormwater." "Of the households contracted, nobody today finds any use for any of the above facilities", says the report.

The water from the wells, say the slum dwellers, is filthy and dirty and without water being available, the baths and latrines cannot be used either. Their old lifestyle for relieving themselves and bathing in open spaces is no worse. Karunanidhi Nagar was just as bad if not a little worse. "In fact, stormwater drains and some parts have even ceased to exist and at other parts mud sand have totally filled them up. The hard surface of the road is barely visible at places and at some places ditches have formed which contained water and dirt" the ORG survey found. The maintenance of TNSCB facilities was to be the responsibility of the Madras Municipal

Corporation. But such a clear division did not materialise. The result, concludes the 1980 survey, "which was observed at the slum level was that though occasionally MMC staff would come for cleaning roads in the areas under their jurisdiction, they would not clean or look to the upkeep of the facilities created by the TNSCB (in the same area)".

Within four years of provision of services, the entire investment had come to nought. The WBIS seems to be relatively better planned and more comprehensive. Part of the multisectoral Madras Urban Development Project-I taken up in 1977-78 under the coordination of the Madras Metropolitan Development Authority (MMDA), the scheme, whose implementation is the responsibility of the TNSCB, is intended to benefit 30,000 households in 36 slums at an average cost of Rs. 1,300 per family. Unlike the EIS the WBIS has standard guidelines, the standard being uniform for all slums. In addition to routine provisions, there is provision for primary and secondary schools, plots for children's creches and sheds providing work space for suitable cottage industries. Preliminary reports indicate that this upgrading project has been significantly more successful than the previous one.

Dharavi, Bombay's and Asia's largest slum, sprawls over 4.5 sq. km. of prime land in Central Bombay. This prime real estate, where huts today fetch a price of Rs. 95,000 was originally creek land, where families of potters and tanners—the Bandra Slaughter House, then existing, was close byhard pitched their shanties. They were soon followed by garbage, rag pickers and scrap dealers and others who brought in their wake common goondas, thugs and slumlords. The encroachers originally occupied private land, but by and by took over municipal as well as government-owned land. Today 2.5 sq. km. of Dharavi land belongs to the Corporation, and one kilometer each to private landowners and the government. Unofficial estimates put the number of shanties, pucca and semi-pucca constructions at over 65,000. The area has a stable population of over 3 lakhs and a floating population of over one lakh, which means that a substantial 4 percent of Bombay lives here.

The slum is a melting pot: 67 percent of the population is Hindu, 26 percent Muslim and the remaining 7 percent divided among the Christians, Sikhs and other minority groups. Though some of Dharavi's 44 clolonies are divided community-wise, most are grouped together by states. Hut sizes vary from 150 sq.ft. huts to over 500 sq. ft. Income groups range from Rs. 400—about 60 percent make this much to those whose earnings could be pegged at anywhere between Rs. 500 and Rs. 1,500 per month and even more. Besides shopowners, a large chunk of Dharavi's population is in government service. It is loosely estimated that over five persons live in a hut, without counting the 'guests' in 'permanent residence'. In addition, the slum dwellers tend to hide their kids, whenever a survey is undertaken, because they think that they will be forcibly sterilised. The average per hut might be as much as eight persons.

Hyderabad's population in 1981 was estimated at 2-2 million of which approximately 500.000 lived in slums. The city's slum dwellers have participated in an urban community development (UCD) project which covered barely 4,000 people in nine slums in 1967 but embraced 400,000 people in 459 slums by 1981. It was adopted in 1974 by the Hyderabad Municipal Corporation as its main policy for slums, and over the period 1974-84 has proved to be a highly successful slum upgrading programme which now covers over 81 percent of the city's slum population.

Hyderabad was one of the 20 cities along with Ahmedabad, Baroda, Calucutta and others, selected in

1967 for a Central Government sponsored series of pilot projects in urban community development. But it is only in Hyderabad that progress was made in converting a successful pilot project into a relatively successful city-wide programme.

The main components have been emphasis on self-help in bringing about and maintaining improved civic amenities; granting of land tenure to the slum residents by the municipal corporation; and a flexible responsive and dedicated approach on the part of the project organisers. The slum dwellers simply determine the location of taps and latrines, the width of the paved passanges and soon. They have contributed in greater measure, with labour and money, to improve housing and build community centres. Each household pays upto 75 percent of rebuilding costs of their home through bank loans.

The slum dwellers also contribute to community centre activities; balwadis (creches), adult literacy classes and cottage industry cooperatives. What made this high degree of involvement and self-help possible was the granting of ownership rights (pattas) to each household for their plot. This not only assured the slum dwellers of the benefits of whatever they invested in rebuilding their homes, it also made it feasible for the city's banks to grant them loans by holding their pattas as mortage. Between 1977 and 1983 the Andhra Pradesh government gave pattas to 13,000 additional households, which enabled 13,000 new houses to be built in various low income areas.

The resident families are far more concerned with maintenance than they would be if the Government had built the houses and handed them over. Moreover out of a total cost of Rs. 9.6 crore, the government has spent only Rs. 1.1 crore. Nationalised banks have advanced loan of upto Rs. 8,00 per household to individuals recommended by the project staff at very low rates of interest, repayable over 20 years. The actual expenditure per house incurred by the people has varied between Rs. 10,000 and Rs. 12,000. The difference between the loaned amount and actual costs has been made up by the people tapping their own and their relatives' resources, by subsidies from the UNICEF at the rate of Rs. 200 per house for private lavatories and by subsidies from local organisation like Lions, Rotary and Jaycees at the rate of Rs. 500 to Rs. 1,000 to cover the costs of reinforced concrete slabs.

Delhi is one of the fastest growing cities of India. The population of the Union Territory has increased from 2.61 million in 1961 to 6.22 million in 1981 and increase of 3.56 million in just 20 years. It is 93.70 lakhs as per 1991 census and is expected to reach 13.26 million by 2001. According to the provisional figures released by the census authorities, Delhi's population in 1991 stood at 93.7 lakhs, an increase of 31.5 lakhs over the 1981 figure. This represents a decadal growth rate of between 50 to 64 percent compared to 53 percent in the previous decade when the city's population increased by 21.5 lakhs. However, the biggest jump was withnessed in the decade 1941-51, when the number really doubled following the influx of refugees from Pakistan.

Despite the concept of NCR, the influx of migrants to Delhi from the neighbouring States continues. The Perspective Plan for Delhi, like its forerunner, the Master Plan, seeks to divert a considerable number of people to towns in the periphery of the city. But as these places lack adequate infrastructure, migrants inevitably make their way to Delhi. The 1981 census, which covered housing conditions too, revealed that only 41 percent of the households in Delhi had roof of concrete RBC/RCC, while 38 percent had roof of stone, bricks, or lime, Twenty-one percent of the households had roof of completely substandard type such as grass, reeds, wood, tiles or slate, corrugated iron sheets or asbestos cement sheets. The census does not categorise the houses into pucca and kutcha houses.

However, for our purposes we have taken those houses as pucca houses which had got floors of cement, bricks, stone and lime and mosaic tiles, combined with walls burnt bricks or stone or cement concrete and roofs made of concrete RBC/RCC. Using this definition, we find that 73 percent of the households in Delhi city lived in pucca houses. Of these, only 40 percent had got roof of concrete, PRC/RCC, 17 percent had got roof of brick, stone and lime and 16 percent had roof of stone only. That is, even using a very liberal definition of pucca houses, roughly one-fourth of the households in Delhi city lived in substandard housing conditions while only 40 per cent of the households lived under RBC/RCC roofs in 1981.

About 4.6 percent of households lived in completely kutcha houses whose floors are made of mud, wood, bamboo etc., walls are made of grass, reeds, mud wood, or G.I. sheets and roofs are made of grass reeds, thatch, tiles, slate/shingles corrugated sheets or asbestos cement sheets. Apart from this, 1.36 percent of the households were found to be houseless. We can look at this from another angle i.e., by the number of rooms occupied by a household. Fifty-four percent of the household lived in one-room accommodation, while 26 percent had two-room houses. Only 18 percent of the households had more than two- room accommodation with them, It was also found that 44 percent of the households living in one-room houses had five or more members in the household while 61 percent of the household living in one-room houses had five or more members in the household while 61 percent of the households living in one-room houses had five or more members in the household while 61 per cent had four or more members in the household.

Populationwise, 48 percent of the population of Delhi lived in one-room houses and 29 percent lived in two-room houses. As for the tenure status of the houses occupied by the household, 51 percent lived in their own houses and 49 percent lived in rented houses. During 1981 cenus, data had also been collected on the availability of drinking water, electricity facilities to the households. Twentyfive percent of the households in Delhi city did not have electricity in their houses, while 32 percent of the households did not have toilet facilities. This is rather appalling.

Among the there municipalities, the position was the worst in Delhi Cantt. areas and the most satisfactory in N.D.M.C. areas. In N.D.M.C. areas, only 7 percent of the population did not have electricity facilities while in M.C.D. Cantt. areas this percentage was 19 and 26, respectively. In respect of toilet facilities, 11 percent of the population in N.D.M.C. areas, 27 percent in M.C.D. and 35 percent in Delhi Cantt. areas did not have them within the premises of their houses.

Only 51 percent of the households in the urban areas of Delhi had access to tap water within their premises, while another 17 percent had access to tap water outside the premises. Some 27 percent of the Households relied on hand pumps or tube wells for drinking water supply. While in N.D.M.C. areas, 84 percent of households had access to tap water within the premises, in Delhi Cantt. areas and M.C.D. areas, this percentage was 69 and 54, respectively. Since about 55 percent of Delhi's growth is attributable to migration largely consisting of literate and semi-literate persons from the rural areas of neighbouring States, the position of housing in Delhi would have become much worse since 1981. To work out the dimensions of the housing problem during 1981-91, we have to add to this the estimated net migrants (16.55lakh) to Delhi during 1981-91 and also that component of the natural increase of Delhi's population in 1981-91 which occurs among the slum-dwellers. Out of this expected natural increase of 14 lakh population, around five lakh can be assumed to occur among those 27 percent of the households of Delhi in 1981 who lived in substandard housing conditions.

In case of electricity and toilet facilities, the data, the percentage of both the households and the population with or without these facilities are available and they are approximately the same, as noted earlier. But in case of housing data and data on water supply, only the percentage of households are available. It is assumed here that these percentages closely approximate the percentage of population also. Thus, the dimensions of the housing problems of Delhi during the decade 1981-91 would be :

(a) Provision of suitable house to 38 lakh persons;

(b) provision of tap drinking water to 40 lakh persons;

(c) provision of electricity to 35 lakh persons;

(d) Provision of toilet facilities to 39 lakh persons.

We have also to take into account that part of the expected natural increase of population which would occur among the population living in good housing conditions, the provision of standard houses, electricity, tap water and toilet facilities to such large populations is a stupendous tasks. The Administration would have to gear itself to this tasks failing which Delhi would have large slums all around the city with its concomitant social, economic and political consequences. Projecting this scenario still further into the next decade, we would be faced with a very staggering picture. Delhi's population is expected to inrease by 40 lakh during 1991-2001, out of which, 23.64 lakh are likely to be due to net in-migration and 16.455 lakh due to natural increase. Adding these 40 lakh persons, the housing targets for 1981-2000 decades would be: (1) provision of housing to 78 lakh persons, (2) provision of tap drinking water to 80 lakh persons, (3) Provison of electricity to 75 lakh persons and (4) provision of toilet facilities to 79 lakh persons. Urbanisation is a conceomitant of economic development and in the economically advanced countries at least, it ensures better life for the inhabitants of the urban areas. In the developing countries, however, the situation is not rosy.

The rapid increase in population of the bigger cities in the developing countries is largely due to a combination of the push and pull factors. Migration of literate and semi-literate economically deprived population from the rural areas to the urban areas in search of employment ends to create a class of people in the urban areas who are both socially as well as economically deprived of the benefits of urbanisation and they tend to live in very poor and shabby conditions. We have already noticed that the housing conditions are pretty bad for at least one-fourth of the households of Delhi. This is true of most of the bigger cities in India as well as in other developing countries. Special attention needs to be paid for provision of cheap housing and other civic amenities to these people, otherwise the modern cities of the third world would become centres of poverty, squalor and disease.

The city's transport system can best be described as 'chaotic' with the motor vehicles choking the roads and polluting the air with their noxious emissions. Furthermore, an average of six people die each day on the roads due to accidents. With 20,000 buses, 10,700 taxi cabs and 77,000 three wheeler scooter rickshaws, the public transport system of Delhi is grossly inadequate to meet the needs of a growing population. Hence, a large number of people are forced to use private vehicles to go to work.

Delhi's vehicle population has grown dramatically during the last decade. The total number of moter vehicles increased by an incredible 13.80 lakh over a ten-year period from 5,92,584 in 1982 to 19,72,998 in 1962. A large percentage of this increase is accounted for by the phenomenal growth in the number of two wheelers from 3.87 lakhs to 13.17 lakhs during the same period. The number of private cars, jeeps and vans also increased from 1.28 lakhs to 4.4 lakhs. The growth in the number of taxis and three wheelers, however, has been significantly slower.

The ambient air quality in Delhi gives it the dubious distinction of being the fourth most polluted city in the world. A major reason for the increase in air pollution is the rising number of motor vehicles and the two coal-based thermal power plants that operate within city limits. Of the total emission load of around 2090 tpd, over 1319.96 tpd are due to automobile exhaust—60 percent of total emissions.

While the levels of sulphur dioxide and oxides of nitrogen are within the prescribed limits, the level of suspended particulate matter (SPM) is extremely high. This is partly due to naturally dusty conditions. But in addition to industries and the power station, as well as stone crushing quarries located on the periphery of the city contribute to the SPM load. Though the thermal power plants do have electrostatic precipitators, which are to reduce the quantity of pollutants discharged into the air, they do not always function efficiently. However, when they do work, the difference is dramatic: the fly ash emitted drops from 800-3000 mg/ nm3. The vehicular pollution level monitored at the ITO crossing in Delhi, essentially a commercial area, over the last few years indicates that the average carbon monoxide presence at this busy traffic junction is well below the industrial area limit of 4.39 ppm but above the 1-75 ppm limit laid for residential area.

The British planned hill stations for their own enjoyment with utmost care. Within independence they were open to more and more people and in recent years the traffic has increased enormously. Ironically, the authorities' ambitious residential schemes and the 'development' of tourist facilities have destroyed neighbouring forests, critically reducing the towns water supply. As a result the hill stations, a haven from the heat and bustle of the plains, are dying.

Acute water shortage is common to most hill resorts. Ootacamund (Ooty) near Bangalore, situated in a district which produced 50% of the State's hydel power, in 1982 faced one of the worst droughts of the century. Darjeeling, a summer time retreat suffers an annual shortage of drinking water. In Panchgani, on Mahabaleshwar's eastern ridge, the forest department is left with a ridiculous 25 hectares of forests and Mahabaleshwar slopes are now more or less totally denuded. As such Vennal lake, only water source for the town is silting up.

Matters are made worse by a tremendous increase in both the permanent population and the tourist traffic. The population of Shillong in 1971 was 1.22 lakh, today it is double. In Shimla, the summer capital of the British, civic facilities have all but collapsed. Every tourist season, one lakh people are added to their swell. Today, it is difficult for natural resources to keep pace with growth. The natural charm of a hill resort has been battered. For instance, in Shillong, instead of towering pines there are rows of houses.

Bangalore, Pune and Dehra Dun were for long praised as idyllic towns, cool green and quiet. Today all three are boom towns, noisy, dusty and hot. Bangalore is one of the 10 fastest growing cities in the world. It was a small village in the 16th century. It grew to an important textile production centre under Tipu Sultan. Under the British the city saw some limited industrial development. Since independence, massive investment in public sector industries has completely changed its character.

Between 1971 and 1981, the city's population exploded by 76 percent from 1.64 million to 2.91 million. Inevitably, the total number of slums grew from 159 in 1972 to 287 in 1982; the slum population grew from 1.31 lakh to about 3 lakh, packed into 3,451 acres or 11 percent of the city corporation areas. By metropolitan standards, Bangalore can still be described almost a slumless city, but the trends are frightening.

The former Punyapur of the 8th century Rashtrakuta kings, where Shivaji once rode his horse, has not fared much better. Pune is today the base of some of the country's biggest industries, and has in the process turned into a giant sprawling along the ribbon typing it to Bombay, with a population of 1.46 million. The number of slums grew from 127 in 1950 to...in 1976.

Dehra Dun has suffered similar changes. The lush green hill resort used to be the preserve of government instiutions like military academies, the Forest Research Institute and the Survey of India. But in 1960s the area was declared industrially backward and conscessions and incentives announced. Since then a large number of quarries and industrial units based on mines produce have come up. Of the 26 major industrial units in Dehra

Dun, 50 percent are limestone based, and 210 small scale crushers are causing serious air pollution problems. The population has grown from 30,0000 to 40,000 in the early 20th century to 0.42 million and is expected to reach 0.6 million by 2000.

The problems that growth has brought in its wake are manifold. Till 1895, Bangalore City got its water from a number of tanks such as Darmambudhi, Sampangi, Ulsoor and Sankey, supplemented by local wells and ponds. Most have been swallowed up and the disturbance in the watershed has accelerated the drying up of tanks in 1925, the Hesarghata lake became alomost dry and today the Sankey tank is one of the few that has not been swallowed up. These miniature lakes also contributed to local cooling.

Many major cities have moved from slum demolition and mass eviction to slum assistance. Self-help is an important ingredient making government intervention in the housing sector more effective. But projects have fallen short of expectations; production of serviced sites is low and they are not accessible to the very poor; slum upgrading has been superficial, of no lasting significance. Land is of central importance. Governments have gone in for vacant, perpheral plots, avoiding the issue of finding lands by means which can be replicated on a large scale.

In slum upgrading projects, and issue, except in Hyderabad, has been avoided altogether. This has had serious consequences: the upgraded house, joint and housing market uncontrolled by the authorities, and the poor can be squeezed out if they can't afford to pay the higher rents, or can be tempted into selling. If the urban poor are to have significantly improved access to upgraded slums and new serviced sites, the government must flood the city's low income housing market with self-help housing stock. Otherwise even the few sections of the urban poor who have benefited from protected pilot projects will soon be displaced by market forces. That this danger can be avoided and real progress made in self-help housing for the urban poor is demonstrated by the case of Hyderabad's upgrading programme which recognised the importance of granting land tenure from the very beginning. At present, government policy wavers between slum improvement and slum bulldozing. There is not clear national plan to give every city dweller a proper roof.

A fundamental choice has to be made. As M.N. Buch argues, either Indians can plan for "a built environment in which every citizen has reasonable access to water, lives in developed lots where drainage is satisfactory and where roads are so designed as to provide efficient and cheap public transport" or "for" one in which there are areas of excellence and other areas of total degradation". If it is accepted that the former choice alone will lead to a better quality of life for the maximum number of people then Indians will have to reconcile themselves to the fact that for years to come our cities will be just a collection of shacks. This means that the perceptions of planners and architects will have to change dramatically. The power of the upper classes, who want to use the cheap labour of slum dwellers but want to deny them a home, will have to be curbed.

4 CAUSES AND IMPACT OF GAS TRAGEDY

The presumption of alternatives—environment or economic growth—goes against the concept of sustainability. Without economic growth, environment cannot be protected; and without environmental protection, economic growth will be non-sustainable. The natural environment in developing countries has the very resources that form the basis for economic growth, and the irreversible damage and misuse of these resources (such as land, air, water, forests, rivers, and lakes) will be the equivalent of eliminating the very base of development.

Union Carbide (India) Ltd. is a subsidiary of Union Carbide Corpn. Inc. (USA). The Bhopal plant of Union Carbide (India) which commenced its operations in 1969 deals with agricultural chemicals. The production of carbaryl pesticides was planned from 1977. Because of some design problems, methyl isocyanate was initially imported from the USA for the manufacture of carbaryl pesticides. MIC production started in the Bhopal plant during 1979. The demand for carbaryl pesticides was less than anticipated, and Union Carbide did not make a profit in the operation of this division. Because of the lack of profit, there was a resistance to incurring additional investments for the safety or modernization of instrumentation. Any safety lacunae have to be viewed against this background.

When the MIC plant was set up, one of the conditions stipulated by Union Carbide Corpn. (UCC) was that the plant should have its own trained superintendent. At the Bhopal plant, MIC was not sold and all the pesticide produced at Bhopal was sold to the Indian market. Methyl isocyanate is a colourless liquid with a powerful odour. The boiling point is 39°C at normal atmospheric pressure and it has a flash point of 7°C below zero. MIC is highly volatile, but stable under dry conditions. It is also highly reactive and gives rise to a number of products ranging from simple carbates to polyurethane formulations such as foams, adhesives, and plastics. MIC is biologically very active; even in very small amounts it causes irritation of the eyes.

When inhaled it reacts vigorously with fluids in the lungs. Since the gases produced are heavy, oxygen is expelled from the lungs, causing choking and even death. Injury to human beings from MIC occurs through two routes, namely, (i) accidental absorption in massive doses, resulting in acute toxicity, and (ii) prolonged exposure to low concentrations of the vapour in the air, leading to chronic toxicity or sensitization of the subjects. The threshold limit value for an 8-hour exposure in air for MIC is 0.02 ppm as per the Union Carbide India manual.

Methyl isocyanate is five times more toxic than the lethal gas phosgene. This is mainly due to the high volatility, high reactivity, low solubility, and high penetration of MIC. MIC reacts with almost all vital bio-substances in the body such as amino acids, ribonuclease, chymotypsin, haemoglobin, and sensitive enzymes, and in many cases inactivates them. Because of this, the toxic effects of MIC can be long-lasting and irreversible. It has been reported that even 90 days after the accident, the concentration of carboxyhaemoglobin and methaemoglobin had not fallen in some of the patients exposed to MIC at Bhopal. MIC polymerizes in the presence of external substances and also reacts with water. To inhibit the polymerization of MIC, phosgene, which reacts with water producing hydrochloric acid, is added while storing.

The possible cause of the Bhopal accident was the accidental entry of water into the MIC tank which must have resulted in the partial removal of the inhibitor (phosgene) and the production of the catalyst (hydrochloric acid). The MIC pipes were being washed just prior to the accidental release of MIC on 2 December 1984. When MIC polymerizes, a large quantity of heat is released. Polymerization of MIC, which is catalyzed by hydrochloric acid, is 200 times faster at 25°C than at 0°C: hence refrigeration is a prime safety precaution. Another reason for the accidental entry of water into the MIC storage tank was a plant modification carried out a year before the accident Water entered through a jumper line which connects the Relief Valve Vent Header (RVVH) and Process Vent Header (PVH). The RVVH and PVH were interconnected mainly to facilitate the removal of MIC. Even if the scrubber or flare unit is disconnected, the MIC released will be vented through it common outlet.

There were thousands of people who became the victims of this gas disaster. Most of them were the city's poor, living in the sprawling settlements opposite and around the Union Carbide factory. One of them is Ramanarayan Jadav, a driver of the city corporation, who says that he had started feeling the gas around 11.30 p.m. itself. But he stayed on for at least another 45 minutes because "this much gas used to leak every eighth day and we used to feel irritation in the chest and in the eyes. But finally everything used to calm down. Even if the company had put off its warning siren then, many could have escaped.

But nothing happened and many thousands woke up only between 12.30 and 1 a.m. by which time the gas was spreading in high concentrations. People woke up coughing violently and with eyes burning as if chilly powder had been flung into them. As the irritation grew and breathing became impossible, they fled, some with their families and many without. They got on to whatever they could—cycles, bullock carts, buses, cars, autorickshaws, tempos, trucks and mopeds. Scooters had whole families on them. Trucks were full but people hung on outside, some grabbing the legs and hands of those already inside. Small children, old men and women were pushed in handcarts or carried. By 3 a.m. the main thoroughfares were jammed with an unending and uncontrollable stream of humanity. The streets were foul with vomit. Those who fell were trampled by the crowd. The worst affected were the children: unable to walk and breathe, they simply suffocated and died.

Thousands fled to towns hundreds of kilometers away Sheore, Vidisha, Hoshangabad, Raisen, Obaidullaganj, Ashta, Ujjain, Dewas, Indore, Ratlam and even Nagpur 400 km away. About 10,000 men, women and children reached Sehore between 2 a.m. and 4 a.m. Another 10,000 went to Raisen. They flocked to the district hospitals for treatment. Hundreds of people who dashed to Ujjain and Indore had to be immediately hospitalised there. In the midst of this frenzy, there was no dearth of valour. Hundreds of taxi, autorickshaw, tempo and turck operators risked their lives to evacuate thousands of people.

The gas that spewed out of the high-tech factory of the multinational Union Carbide spread over some 40 sq. km. and affected people seriously as distant as 5 km to 8 km downwind. For nearly 200,000 people, a quarter of the city's population, Bhopal became a gas chamber. If it were not for the two lakes of Bhopal which came in the way of gas cloud and neutralised.

Exactly what happened in the Union Carbide factory that night is still not known officially from the Government of India. But press reports have built up the following sequence of events. MIC is stored in three double-walled, partly buried stainless steel tanks—code named 610,611 and 619. While thousands slept in their huts around the pesticide factory on the night of December 2/3 a skeleton staff of 120 workers inside the factory ended its shift round 10.45 p.m. and a new shift took over around 12 p.m.

One of the workers then noticed that the pressure in tank 610—the tank from which all the MIC finally escaped—had risen from the 2 lb square inch (psi), recorded by the earlier shift, to around 10 psi. Corresponding tank temperatures were not available as they were not logged normally. The fivefold increase in pressure within an hour was dismissed in the belief that the pressure recording instrument could be faulty. Shakil Qureshi, the supervisor on duty, said later, "Instruments often didn't work. They got corroded. Crystals would form on them". At about 11.30 p.m. workers in the plant realised there was an MIC leak somewhere when their eyes began to fear.

A few of them walked around the MIC structure and spotted a drip or liquid about 50 feet off the ground and some yellowish-white gas accompanying the drop. They told Qureshi about the leak of about 11.45 p.m. Qureshi however decided to deal with the leak after the tea break, scheduled for 12.15 a.m. Qureshi says he was told only of a water leak. But by the time the tea break ended at 12.40 a.m. events were moving very fast.

Suman Dey, a worker at the plant noticed that the temperature gauge on tank 610 had reached 25°C, the top of its scale, and pressure was rapidly moving towards 40 psi, the point at which the emergency relief valve opens,

He rushed to the storage tanks to investigate and was horrified. As he stood on a concrete slab above the storage tanks, the slab suddenly began to shake. "There was to tremendous sound," a messy boiling sound underneath the slab, like a cauldron". He ran, only to hear a loud noise behind him.

The slab made of 60 feet of concrete, at least 6 inches thick was cracking. The heat was like a blast-furnance. He couldn't get within six feet of it. He then heard a loud hissing sound and saw gas shoot out of a tall stack connected to the tank and form a white cloud drifting over the plant and towards the sleeping neighbourhood in the plant, he found that the pressure indicator had gone above 55 psi, the top of the scale, and the safety valve had opened releasing MIC from the storage tank.

UCC's report on incident claims that the tank had 90,000 pounds of MIC at the time of the incident. For approximately two hours the safety valve remained open releasing over 50,000 pounds of MIC in vapour and liquid—and goodness alone knows what other gases phosgene, hydrogen cyanide. Carbon dioxide, oil of which have been mentioned. Sometimes between 1.30 a.m. and 2.30 a.m the safety valve reseated, as the tank pressure went below 40 psi.

The plant has two main safety devices. The first is a scrubber, which neutralises the gas caustic soda if the scrubber fails, the gas goes to the flare tower to be burnt off. Both the safety systems failed to work that night. For days, newspapers reported guesses about why the safety systems did not work. On December 7, the first real big news appeared. Leaders of the factory employees' union claimed that the vent gas scrubber had been under repair. About 10 days later, the factory Works Manager, J Mukund publicly contradicted this report but was unable to answer how he knew the vent scrubber had worked.

UCC has since claimed that the used caustic soda tank was hot to touch (60°C) on the morning of December 3, indicating that it must have worked. But if is now also widely accepted that the scrubber was grossly under-designed and could not have neutralised more than a fraction of escaping gases. The flare did not work because the management had disconnected the pipleline running from the vent scrubber to the flare tower for maintenance and connected it to a vent gas pipe which went straight to the atmosphere. Even the flame on the flare tower had been shut off. Thus, all the plant's safety devices were down.

There were three other safety systems that were either not used that night or proved to be underdesigned. First, the factory has a network of water jets, but they could not reach the height at which the MIC was gushing into the air. Second, the MIC storage tanks are connnected to a 30 tonne refrigeration system which keeps liquid MIC at 0°C. The refrigeration system has been closed down in June 1984, and the gas was at 15 — 20°C. Had the refrigeration system been working or capable of working, the MIC could have been cooled. Refrigeration would have increased the time available for the detection of the chemical reaction and safe disposal of the material before the reaction reached a dangerous speed. Third, the Bhopal plant had three tanks, each with a 60 tonne capacity, one of which was to be always kept empty for contingencies. But all the tanks contained MIC that night.

But what caused the violent reaction that night? Union Carbide's scientists have been aware of the possibility of an explosive 'runway reaction' in MIC. This gas can react with almost any chemical, including itself, to generate substantial quantities of heat and carbon dioxide. The heat released causes the reaction to speed up, which generates more heat, and pressure can thus go on building until it finally reaches an explosive level. The longer the MIC sits in storage tanks, the greater the chance of side-reactions building up to a runaway reaction.

The MIC at the Bhopal plant had been sitting in the storage tank since October. Demand for carbaryl was not very high. The precise sequence of events still remains obscure. Carbide's report has claimed that it was a unique combination of large amounts of water (120 to 240 gallons), higher than normal amounts of chloroform in the stored MIC (several per cent instead of a maximum of 0.5 per cent), and an iron catalyst, that lead to the violent reaction in MIC, stored at a higher than specified temperature in the tank. Simultaneously, MIC got polymerised, the reaction being catalysed by iron resulting from the corrosion of the tank walls due to the high temperatures. Carbide claims that the corrosion rate increased markedly because of the presence of an abnormaly high level of chloroform. The rapid release of carbon dioxide in large quantities then helped to build up high pressures, which forced the foaming mass of chemicals out of tank.

By the time the sun rose, hundreds, some even say thousands, lay dead, many on the roads and many at home under their rattered quilts: corpses with distended bellies were beginning to rot, attracting vultures and dogs. Another 2000 lay dying in hospitals and homes. An equally hideous sight was that of the carcasses of hundreds of dead cattle and animals all over the gas-affected area, swollen up to size of elephants. By about 1 p.m. about 25,000 people were crammed into Hamidia Hospital. The floor was splattered with blood and vomit, Said a doctor at Hamidia : "I was standing in the paediatric department. There was such a terrible crowd, that there wasn't even place to keep bodies on the floor. As soon as a patient was declared, dead his relatives would just vanish with the body. I saw at least 50 bodies taken away like this, I would estimate that anything between 500 and 1,000 bodies were taken away before their deaths could be registered." It was difficult even to distinguish between dead and half-dead bodies. People at the mortuary were unable to cope with and conduct postmortems. One father cried. "They have taken away my son. He was only three years old. My father, mother and two children are in a serious condition. May Allah punish those scoundrels."

The death drama continued for four days. Thousands continued to pour into the hospitals of Bhopal, as some 500 doctors and supporting staff rushed in from other cites of Madhya Pradesh. This is how a foreign correspondent, who reached the city 30 hours after the leak, described the state of gas affected Bhopal: "At the factory, dead bodies were still on the ground, being picked up and loaded aboard a waiting truck. Everywhere one turned, people were retching, racked by violent coughing. All the shops in the city were closed, and on every street people were lying in the gutters. They were dead, humped in agonised frozen postures, like birds short form the sky. In their midst were real birds, vultures. When the vultures swoodped away, the dogs would charge in and tear off pieces of flesh. Resuing the dead from the predators were rifle-toting soldiers of the Indian army, joined by volunteer vigilantes carrying long staves.

Little children with haunted, running, swollen eyes fold of scampering through the night, with no particular destination. They asked the soldiers where they could find their parents. The soldiers replied. 'Wait here' A truck will be along and take you to the hospital. Everyone will be there. The frightened children waited. When the truck came, it took the children to Hamidia Hospital. The army was there too, keeping the human traffic flowing without the usual pushing and shaving. The troops had set up 60 tents, which became instant wards for 20 people each. Some distance away, the army had set up a morgue to which the patrols in the city brought the dead to be identified. The third day saw another 400 deaths at the city's hospitals, which said that 75,000 people had been treated by then. Fresh cases of MIC poisoning continued to arrive, raising fears of after-effects. Some victims showed signs of paralysis, 500 developed corneal ulcers and doctors said that they could go blind. At the burial ground, people helping to dig graves were exhausted, "We are sick of burying the bodies. There is no space" they said.

On the sixth day there way yet another scare. Some 51 fresh cases who had earlier been sent home after being treated for minor eye ailments had to be rushed to the hospitals in a serious condition. Doctors believed that these people may have been affected by the fish eaten from the Bhopal lake. The main fish market of the city was immediately sealed off by the authorities as a precautionary measure. The next day the government announced that slaughter houses were being closed down so that the meat of gas-affected animals could not be sold but there was no ban on the sale of fish. On the seventh day a fresh panic over the disposal of the remaining gas struck the city.

Even as hospital admissions and deaths began to show a steady downward trend the seventh day after the disaster brought a new source of panic to the city; there were still 15 tonnes of the deadly gas left in the factory, which had to be disposed off before Bhopal could really feel safe.

The government entrusted the task of deciding the disposal process to a team of senior scientists headed by Dr. S. Varadarajan, Director-General of the Council of

Scientific and Industrial Research (CSIR). Varadarajan set up his office in the Central Government's Regional Research Laboratory at Bhopal and shrouded himself in complete secrecy, nerve-wracking for the rest of the city.

Journalists were told that there were four ways of disposing off the gas; neutralise it with a chemical like caustic soda (as is expected to happen in the factory's flare tower), pack it into drums and ship it off to the parent Union Carbide in the US or elsewhere, or simply start up the factory and turn it into the factory's final product, the pesticide carbaryl. It was obvious that the company was pushing hard for the last option. Union Carbide Corporation of the US had immediately recommended to its units across the world: use up the reaming MIC to produce carbaryl before governments move in to stop those plants.

The local Union Carbide management had reportedly tried to reopen the plant on December 7 itself, just four days after the tragedy, to dispose off the remaining gas. But the staff which reported for duty was turned back by the district administration in control of the plant. Starting the plant again would mean that the Chief Minister who had previously declared on the fourth day of the disaster that the plant would never be allowed to open again, would have to eat his words. 'The Times of India' pointed out angril, this would amount to a "form of capitulation to the company responsible for the death of over, 1,300 persons...It would tantamount to granting Union Carbide some sort of safety approval or certificate and to letting its management with its all-to-visible safety record, run the plant as it likes".

Word spread on December 10 that the factory had started up again, with one district official claiming that the work to "neutralise the gas had begun" by converting the deadly gas into finished products, but this was immediately denied in a press statement by Varadarajan. The city meanwhile waited tensely. The next day, aimed reports that Varadarajan's teams had restarted the plant for a test run, Arjun Singh appealed to the people: "There is no cause of panic and I repeat there is no reason to evacuate the city." But even so the Chief Minister was saying there was no reason to evacuate the city, he and his government were acting differently.

Government vehicles went around the city announcing to a surprised public that all schools and colleges were being immediately closed for 12 days from the next day. The Madhya Pradesh State Road Transport Corporation admitted to journalists that a large number of buses had been summoned to Bhopal from other parts of the state but clarified that this had been done only to cater to the extraordinary rush of people "returning to Bhopal"!

Regardless of what people thought, the government team began preparations for ensuring extra safety during the disposal process. Experts finally came up with, as they described it to eager newspaper reporters, a six-step safety system. The first step was, in fact, no safety system; it was simply the process by which the pesticide carbaryl is produced by reacting the deadly gas with alphanaphthol.

The second was the standard vent scrubber in the factory that had earlier failed to work. The only addition to this system was a set of fire hozes kept on two sides of the scrubbr to keep it cool in case too much gas came into the scrubber and the reaction with caustic soda increased its temperature. The third safety system was again the standard flare tower. The three new systems that were devised by the experts were based on the high propensity of MIC to react with water, but their flimisiness and simplicity drew much comment. The first of these consisted of a trapaulin shamiana that covered the chimney through which the MIC escapes. This shamiana was to be kept constantly wet, sc that any escaping gas, which did not get burned by the flare tower, would react with water and get converted to harmless dimethyl urea.

The second system consisted of jute mattings hung up on the perimeter wall of the factory on the side of the worst-hit colony on December 3, Jayaprakash Nagar. These too were to be kept wet so that any escaping gas could react with water. The sixth safety system consisted of Indian Air Force helicopters hovering over the plant which could spray water on the escaping gas if needed. If despite all this, immediate evacuation became necessary, people would be warned through sirens and army units, kept on five minutes notice, would move into help.

The jute mattings in particular attracted much derisive comment. Said Praful Bidwai: "There is a length of flimsy jute sacking fastened just over a short stretch of the boundary wall, which is grandiosely termed 'Safety System Five'. The sacking, ruffling in the wind, does not reach belong 12 ft. or 15 ft. from the ground level, a rather low altitude for trapping the gas in case there is an accidental release. Infact, the leading gas, the authorities have presumed without any basis, will also move in a very definite direction and it is not necessary (or, as Dr. Varadarajan says 'possible') to mount the sacking along the entire perimeter wall of the factory."

But three weeks later, there were again fears of outbreaks of epidemics as millions of green flies, attracted by improperly disposed of carcasses, invaded the city. The army had initially helped in the removal and disposal of animal carcasses but the authorities admitted that all the animals could not be buried because of a shortage of sanitary workers and scavengers. Most of the local municipal staff had been affected by the gas and sanitary workers had to be summoned from other towns. Equally disorganised and callous was the administration's response to people's queries. The government began to put out news bulletins over All India Radio on the second day itself that the situation was fast returning to normal and that everything was safe, which, journalists told the chief minister, sounded much like the pronouncements of Carbide officials. The people were suspicious about the air they breathed, the water they drank, and the meat, flour, fish, vegetables they ate. They wanted to know whether dead animals would to an epidemic, weather any gas remained in the factory and whether it could leak out again.

People expressed their growing resentment in various ways. Youth in various gas-affected localities began to gherao medical teams. Less than 100 days after the disaster, an 'Economic times' reporter was taken to houses by angry youth to assess the situation for himself. "Almost every house gave the appearance of a hospital ward," he said in his report "Almost everybody was coughing constantly, having pain and irritation in the chest. Nobody had turned up to provide these people with medicines or to examine them for the last two to three days.

Many of the sick people were not in a position even to get up from bed. Most of them are daily wage earners. They were to getting anything to eat. They had no resources to purchase foodgrains, the women were not physically fit to cook their meals. The moment they were near the fire, their coughing increased. These people generally belong to an economic class which suffers from malnutrition. If they are denied meals in such a shattered physical condition, they would have no resistance left." On December 9 there was even a demonstration in front of the Chief Minister's residence.

Most of the affected people were poor, manual daily wage workers an they found themselves suffering from the effects of MIC even weeks after the exposure the chief one being persistent breathlessness. Manual labour become possible; they felt dizzy even walking one kilometre in the sun. And out of work and money, they found themselves even more diseased, week and hungry, virtually on the verge of starvation. The entire episode left the survivors, their health and their economy totally shattered. Describing a typical situation, a 30-year-old handcart puller Sabir Ahmed said that he had ventured out to work nearly three weeks after the gas leak. But this readearner of a five-member family had to return home soon feeling ill. Porter Bilal Ahmed was in a similar situation, He had received treatment on December 3 at Hamidia Hospital but nothing after that. And he was still experiencing irritation in the eyes, chest pain and nausea, and was finding it impossible to work. Shravan Singh, 34, a lathe operator, now found his earlier occupation which used to fetch him some Rs. 25 a day, so tiring that he had to turn to selling roasted gram as a pavement hawker, earning less than Rs. 10 a day to feed his family of four.

Women often found themselves in a worse situation. They continued to be plagued by blinding headaches, dizziness and could not focus on anything for long. Cooking before the fire brought about exposure to woodsmoke and increased the irritation in their eyes, making impossible to cook more than two chappatis at a time. Bringing water from the nearby well or tap tired them out for the whole day. Many women had lost their sons and husbands and now it was impossible for them to survive, especially as they could not work in their deseased condition. Many of the women living in J.P. Nagar opposite Union Carbide, are bidi workers. Said one bidi worker: "We cannot see the bidi thread after a while; our eyes burn. And Unless you make a sizeable number of bidis and sell them each day, there is no profit." Some bidi workers found that the person who used to purchase bidis from them was dead and therefore there was nobody to sell bidis to even if they could make bidis. The mass death of animals like buffaloes also meant hardship for many people who had lost their sole occupation.

In a desperate bid to get themselves cured, people sat in long queues before mobile clinics, dispensaries and polyclinics set up by the government, and a dozen other dispensaries set up by voluntary agencies. At these centres, they got the same treatment, antibiotics and a few other drugs, which after a while began to create more side-effects than benefits. Those unable to bear their health problems tried to seek the assistance of the big hospitals but from there they were invariably turned back. Other simply lay at home in bed. But with the government and the medical community in Bhopal arguing in less than a fortnight that the worst was over, that most of the problems people were now complaining about were mainly the result of common diseases like anaemia, and TB, rempant in the slums. The people found themselves caught between callers multinational and an inefficient administration system.

The Bhopal disaster has raised a series of questions: Where have other hazardous plants been built in India? Why were so many people living so close to the plant in Bhopal? How do we develop a policy for seeting hazardous factories? Do adequate health and safety laws exist, which might prevent the occurrence of another disaster? Is it true that the benefits of using pesticides are so great that it costs in human lives are outweighted by the lives saved by pesticide use? Do multinationals operate with lower standards for health and safety in their Third World plants than in their home country? Underlying these are deeper issue, about the controls that should govern the industrialisation process, about who decides, whose needs are met by industrialisation, and how multinational corporations, in particular, can be held accountable. Indian newspaper editorials and articles, especially the big English language newspapers, have largely demanded legal controls and regulations. They have pointed out the inadequacies of the air and water pollution control laws, laws like the Factories Act which are supposed to control occupational health problems and oversee safety measures, and laws meant to regulate the use of pesticides.

A carefully screened register of hazardous chemicals and industries is needed. In France, all companies and installations which can pose a danger to the environment have to get themselves registered by law. stronger laws together with stricter implementation have been demanded almost unifromly. Considerable attention has also been given to the seeting of hazardous industries. Western commentators have repeatedly asked why were so many people allowed to live so close to the hazardous plant. The area was uninhabited when the plant was built. Most Indian editorial writers also recommended that hazardous industries be set up far away from populated areas.

The Central Board for the Prevention and Control of Water and Air Pollution has recommended unihabited green belts 2-3 km in all directions around hazardous industries. One newspaper writer suggested that this 12-30 sq. km. green area could "either be sold to the concerned companies at a low rate (for experimental farms, etc.) or be kept with the state local government". As for slums, which already exist around hazardous industries, it has been demanded that they be removed forthwith. This view that people, not industries, need to be removed, has been enchoed by numerous industrialists since the disaster.

A third point concerns imported chemicals. A number of pesticides and drugs banned or heavily restricted elsewhere are being knowingly imported or manufactured in India. An example is polychlorinated biphenyls (PCBs), used in electrical capacitors and transformers. PCBs have been banned in most developed countries because they produce cancer. In many small scale industries where these chemicals are used, workers are not even conscious of the danger. The fourth point made is about the choice of technology. For instance, many companies manufacture carbaryl without using MIC and, indeed, Union Carbide itself switched to using MIC only a decade before the Bhopal plant was licensed.

Industrial licensing authorities made no attempt to assess the advantages of the alternative route in Indian conditions. They seem to have been carried away with Carbide's offer to bring the latest technology. On the contrary, France refused to allow MIC to be produced. A caprolactam plant uses the same hazardous process used at Flixborough in UK, when suffered one of worst fires known to chemical industry in 1974, when cyclohexane vapour was released. A safer alternative process could have been used.

A fifth point relates to the transportation of toxic chemicals. MIC was being transported from Bhopal to several locations in India without any regulations. Nearly 100 accidents involving release of toxic chemicals during rail transport occur in the US every year. Two accidents on an average involve damages of over a million dollars. Since Bhopal tragedy, local communities and states in the US have begun passing restrictions regarding transport of substances like MIC. They have refused to wait for adequate federal regulations.

A sixth point takes in the behaviour of multinational corporations, which have repeatedly exported banned drugs and pesticides and even entire factories to the Third World, Asbestos today is the largest single cause of occupational cancer in the US, and experts have calculated that 8000 to 10,000 Americans will die annually over the next 20 years because of exposure to absestos in the past. Use of asbestos in industrial nations has declined precipitiously—in Britain, by 52 per cent between 1975 and 1982 and in the US, by 60 per cent from 1971.

Sweden has virtually eliminated the use of asbestos, the result of a trade union campaign since 1975. But cement materi:ls is growing. In Ahmedabad, Shree Digvijay Cement produces 50,000 tonnes of asbestos-cement pipes and sheets per year. Its foreign collaborator, John Manvile Corporation, was so heavily sued in the US that it took refuge under bankruptcy laws. In Bombay, Hindustan Ferrodo, in collaboration with the British company, Turner and Newall, manufactures asbestos textiles and brake linings, which are being abandoned in Europe and USA. No attempt has been made by these companies to inform Indian workers or consumers of the dangers of abestos.

All these suggestions pose serious problems. Take, or instance, the idea of seeting hazardous industries away from human habitation. Zoning is relatively successful in Western countries, where an affluent population has access to efficient transport facilities. By contrast, a sizeable fraction of India's urban population cannot afford even subsidised public transport system. Moreover, Western cities have never faced the kind of rapid growth that Third World cities face today.

Slums come up where work opportunities exist, and usually at such a speed that urban planners find them extremely difficult to control. Industrialisation and urbanisation go hand in hand. Industries immediately become focal points for urban growth and accretion of settlements. In fact, many chemical plants even in the United State, are situated in crowded uraban areas, in particular older plants which came up during the Second World War and before. Union Carbide's other MIC-producing plant at Institute, West Virginia, is a prime example. A siting policy which pushes hazardous industries into 'backward' rural area could easily become an excuse for displacing rural people.

Workers in remotely located plants will also need transport facilities. Unless Indians want to blame the victims for the suffering caused by such disaster, the country must realise that it has only two options for hazardous industries: either such industries are not built at all by adopting suitable technology or lifestyle choices, or if they have to be built, they will have to live cheek by jowl with people (especially poor people), in which case safety measures must overroide all considerations, including economic considerations. And to ensure that safety measures are indeed undertaken, the people must be fully involved about all possible dangers.

Indian social action groups strongly argued for the people's right to know about hazardous factories, where they are being side, why and what dangers they pose. Only when people know will there be public pressures for safety and a honest response from regulators. The callousness with which the warnings about the Bhopal plant were ignored shows an unholy politician-industrialists nexus operating in full bloom.

Several commentators have also raised broader questions about the very pattern of industrialisation, which generates such a massive demand for toxic substances and which exposes the poor to such hazards. Western newspapers have quickly reminded the Third World about 'a balance sheet of death' as the 'Guardian' in London put it, or 'The pain of progress', as the 'New York Times' put it. Said the pro-industry Wall Street Journal: "Of the people killed, half would not have been alive if it were not for that plant and the modern health standards made possible by the use of pesticides". The British science magazine "New Scientist", has been equally pointed in its remarks: 'Rich nations can afford to forego a little pesticide for fear of spreading a rare cancer. Such arguments mean little in countries where thousands die from hunger. Thus, if pesticides kill they also save'.

In any case, many multinational executives have asked, why should developed countries be responsible for controls on products used by developing countries? Would't that be a kind of 'environmental imperialism'? James Weeks, a commentator in consumer crusaders, Ralph Nader's Multinational Monitor has argued back. "This concern obscures a more fundamental issue: the dictating that is already being done by an international economic system dominated by the same multinationals." In 1981, President Ronald Reagon overturned an executive order by former President James Carter to inform developing countries about export of products banned in the US, because it could affect US exports.

India's ruling elite probably believes in the 'balance sheet of death' argument. Commenting on the fact that hardly any English newspaper had criticised the Industrialisation process itself, one Hindi poetess lamented: "there was no anger in any of the newspapers".

There were indeed only a few exceptions. Said Perahash Johsi, the editor of Jansatta: "The bnefits of 21st of 21st century technology will go to politicians, administratiors, scientists and so-called intellectuals. But the people who have to pay the price of this technology with their lives are those who cannot even get enough to eat two times a day. Borrowed technology from the west cannot fill the gap between these two worlds. This guilt is beyond the understanding and resolution power of the West". The Zahreeli Gas Sangarsh Morcha and several voluntary groups across the country have demanded an alternative development process, which will be based not only on appropriate technological choices, but also on appropriate life style choices.

There is no particular reason, for instance, why there should be such a demand for plastics, detergents or polyurethane foam. The demand for these products has arisen out of aggressive marketing policies, whose sole interest is to increase corporate profits. In agriculture too, there is no real need to rely heavily on pesticides. While insecticide use has increased 11-fold over the past 30 years, crop losses due to insect resistance doubled.

Through land reforms, soil conservation measures, building of small water harvesting systems like traks and ponds, planting of multipurpose food, fuel and fodder tree species, intercropping and use of resistant crop varieties, setting up of integrated systems of animal husbandry, crops, orchards and aquaculture, villages can be turned into highly productive, symbiotically integrated ecosystems of food-fish-fertiliser-fodder biomass, and the need for chemical fertilizers and pesticides can be almost eliminated.

In the area of public health, India's own scientific laboratories have shown that the town of Pondicherry and villages of Gujarat can get rid of mosquitoes by policies that help the people to clean up their environment. What is the value of dumping more powerful insecticides while mosquitogenic, filthy conditions are being simultaneously created for mosquito-brone diseases to grow? But a move away form highly toxic, bulldozing chemicals will require a holistic approach to people's problems and people's participation in the management of national resources and generation of technology. This will come about only, as poet Raghubir Sahay has put it, with a culture of anusandhan (research and discovery) and not one of anukaran (blind imitation).

Several commentators have been extremely pessimistic about such a culture actually being born. They argue that this culture based on modern technology is so seductive that changing it will be extremely difficult task. Asked one writer from Bhopal; we may be able to stop the multinational corporation from coming in but can we stop the 'multinational culture'? Is the not the culture that all of us crave for? "As if to prove his point, there was no effect of the Bhopal dissaster on the fortunes of the ruling party in the parliamentary elections from Madhya Pradesh.

The ruling party also won the seat of Bhopal. Said Rajkumar Keshwani, the journalist who had given warning of the disaster two years before: "I don't see any anger. I only see shattered people. And outside the affected areas, there is only a desire of more of the same." Five months later, the government still had not taken any steps to prevent the recurrence of Bhopal-type disasters. A proposal to set up an inter-mnisterial board on hazardous chemicals had been quietly buried. The Ministry of Chemicals announced the establishment of a cell, but that too, had not taken off. The Department of Environment was waiting for the Scientific Advisory Committee to the Cabinet to discuss its proposal for a comprehensive Toxic Substance Act. Only some state pollution control boards have started flexing their muscles, basking in all the public attention that they were getting after Bhopal. But what impact their newfound power will have is still not clear.

The Bhopal accident identifies a number of issues. In many instances the failure to adhere to the correct safety factors is nothing but negligence on the part of plant managers. When MIC production started in 1979 at Bhopal the incorporation of the latest safety equipment and monitoring devices should have been ensured. Even if the subsididary did not request for the latest safety systems, the parent company should have insisted on their installation. Further, allowing the manufacturing plant to be situated very close to a growing city, permitting the plant to expand its activities in 1977, allowing squatter settlements to develop close to the factory and subsequently regularizing these illegal occupations, neglecting the safety aspects in spite of six accidents since 1979, and permitting storage of large quantities of MIC indicate that safety was given low priority in government and industry circles.

The safety aspects should be rigorously reviewed in all major factories dealing with hazardous or toxic substances in India. Efforts should be made to claffify hazardous and toxic substances, and a third party safety review for highly hazardous and toxic substance should be made statutory. Industries dealing with hazardous materials should be sited away from human settlements, and existing units should, if necessary, be relocated. Under the existing practice, cities are expanding horizontally and the industrial zones established earlier are getting enguled by human settlements. There should be a long term industrial location policy and plan. Broad zones have to be delineated for setting up different types of industries—polluting, non-polluting, hazarous, and non-hazardous.

The Bhopal accident clearly indicates that there is urgent need for accepted procedures for dealing with transnational enterprise liability. In a period of increasing international contacts, including wide ranging operations by multinational corporations, it is clearly unsatisfactory that the legal mechanisms available to deal with major problems on the transnational level should be restricted by a state system that reflects notions of national sovereignty and autonomy more appropriate to be bygone age.

The world over there is rethinking on the practices of multinational enterprises. It is becoming apparent that it is not only the Third World that has an interest in controlling the activities of multinationals and protecting its citizens from their failings. In the long run, ecologically desirable alternatives such as biological pest control should be attempted. For this purpose, a directional thrust to research in this area has to be attempted. By using genetic enginerring, biotechnology, and biological pest control in a synergistic way we may be able to get away from the chemical pesticies.

5 Environmental Hazards

The principal emissions given off by the chemical industry are gases and vapours of organic chemical compounds such as hydrocarbons and their halogen derivatives, aldehydes, ketones, carboxylic acids, and nitrogen and sulfur compounds (amines, mercaptans, disulfides); gases and vapours of inorganic chemical compounds such as hydrogen sulfide, hydrochloric acid, fluorine compounds, sulfur dioxide, and hydrogen phosphides: and finally toxic powders such as fluorides and carbides, and powders from iron alloys, arsenic and absestos.

Extensive control is necessary, partly because the human sense of smell is very sensitive to substances emitted by chemical industries (such as hydrogen sulfide and mercaptans), even when they are highly rarefied. Thiophenol, for instance, is still perceptible to the human sense of smell in concentrations as low as 1 : 10 billion. To eliminate these substances, purification plants of a very high degree of efficiency are required. Furthermore, the chemical reactions take place in many cases under very heavy pressure.

For safety reasons the reaction apparatuses and accessories must therefore be equipped with pressure-relief facilities (safety valves). In the event of breakdowns, which can be fairly frequent in a chemical works, the noxious substances are released in relatively large quantities. Through the safety valve and connecting attachments of the pipelines, pumps and storage tanks, etc., a multiplicity of small potential outlets are created, the sealing of which in the face of all contingencies cannot be guaranteed. Owing to the large number of noxious chemical substances in existence and the rapid changes that occur in chemical production, the over-all technical development of specific filter appliances to meet all requirements is very hard to achieve.

Altogether the state of air purification technology in the chemical industry is thoroughly unsatisfactory. This is the more serious in that by 1985 the chemical industry reckons on an increase in turnover to about 3.2 times the level in 1970. A particularly sharp rise in production is planned for the sectors that affect the environment most seriously. These sectors, with figures in parentheses showing the average annual production increase planned by 1985, are crop protection and pest destruction agents (3.9%), plastics (4.1%), mineral and coaltar dyes (3.4%), man-made fibers (4.8%), pharmaceuticals (3.6%), etc.

So far, improvements in the discharge of chemicals have been achieved mainly in the field of inorganic production. By the adoption of a new process for sulfuric acid production, the discharge of sulfur dioxide has been reduced by about 80% in relation to conventional production methods. This new technology was introduced not least because it has commercial advantages from the point of view of sulfur recovery.

The petroleum industry is characterized by the regular discharge of hydrocarbons and other organic compounds and of sulfur dioxide and fine dust. Crude oil imported from the oil producing countries is processed in refineries into various petroleum products, in particular heating oil and gasoline. In the refining process, the crude oil is heated and vaporized and then condensed again at various temperatures. In this way the varying fractions, from highly volatile gasoline to heavy heating oil, are separated. In the process, tarlike bituman is left behind for further processing in its turn.

In order to produce the energy needed to vaporize the crude oil, the distillation residues are used in the refineries as the main fuel. These residues contain large quantities of sulfur, which, after combustion, is given off into the atmosphere in the form of sulfur dioxide. In addition, according to where it comes from, the material consumed can contain larger or smaller quantities of fine dust, which is also given off with the flue gas. The second group of components in air pollution by refineries are organic substances such as hydrocarbons. These are discharged in the main from various sources, a ground level, spread over the entire area of the works, such as storage tanks, flanges, safety valves, vents, seals, settling tanks and torch flares. These organic gases and fumes are in some cases very pungent, and so can cause serious nuisance in the vicinity of the refinery.

Between 0.4% and 1% of the crude oil put through a refinery is given off in the form of organic vapours into the environment. Assuming it to have been no more than 0.4%, direct discharges of organic gases and vapours from leaky pipelines and valves come to about 0.08%, the process gases of the torch flares to about 0.23%, and the heating gases of the torch flares and the discharges from the waste water treatment to 0.02% each. On the average the torch has a combustion efficiency rate of no more than 50%—70%. This gives an average discharge rate of organic gases and vapours of 4.3 tons per day per million tons annual average crude oil through put for the refinery. It is assumed at present that one-third of production losses by the petroleum industry pass into the atmosphere as hydrocarbons. An important source of losses is the storage tank. This is best shown by an example: At a temperature of 20°C (68°F) benzene has a vapour pressure of 75 milibars. This represents a saturation density of 320 g per cu m.

When a benzene tank with a capacity of 100,000 cu m is filled at this temperature, with a fixed-top tank, and assuming that only half the saturation density is achieved, about 1.6 tons of benzene will be discharged in the processs. When instead of the fixed-top tank a floating top tank or a fixed-top tank with a floating cover is used, the discharge will drop to about 300 kg of benzene. Discharges into the environment also occur when finished products are loaded into vehicles and vessels for distribution. Each time gasoline is loaded into a container or tanker for transport by land or sea, gas vapour will be discharged into the atmosphere with the expelled air to the amount of about 1.3% of the gasoline transported. The situation is very similar in the case of petrochemistry.

Petrochemial production plants are usually situated in close proximity to refineries, and in them the end products from the refineries are processed further. The petrochemical plants also contain extensive pipeline systems and numerous valves and flanges through which hydrocarbons and other organic compounds are discharged. It is estimated that on the average some 1% of the substances processed in petrochemistry escape in the production process.

A good example of serious irreversible damage to the environment caused by an industrial product which was previously regarded as neutral in its effects is the spray gun, which is in increasing use today for a variety of purposes. As a propellant, the spray gun contains chlorofluorocarbons (CF_2Cl_2 and $CFCl_3$). When the spray gun is used, the propellants are released into the atmosphere. Until recently it was believed that the compounds were so stable that they would not be absorbed or reduced by either plants, soil or water. They were consequently regarded as harmless. In 1974, however, American scientists at the University of Michigan discovered that chlorofluorocarbons could cause serious disturbances in the environment.

The gas rises into the stratosphere and damages the ozone belt surrounding the earth; the ozone belt intercepts a large part of the ionizing radiation coming in from outside and so reduces damage to the earth by this radiation. The process goes as follows. The chlorofluorocarbon molecules are broken down by the strong ultraviolet radiation in the stratosphere. In this way chlorine atoms are released, which break down ozone molecules by a catalytic process (see diagram). The chlorine atom itself is not affected by the process, and in course of time it can split any number of ozone molecules. It is assumed that some 10^{31} ozone molecules per second are broken down in this way today.

The diagram indicates three results of these investigations. In case 1 it is assumed that the use of spray guns and the consequent release of chlorofluorocarbons will go on increasing in the future at the same rate as today. The disintegration rate of the ozone belt, which has been fairly low hiteherto, will then increase sharply after 1980, and this can result in considerable damage on the earth's surface (increase in cancer rate). For Case 2 it is assumed that use of spray guns will increase until 1975 and will remain constant thereafter at the level for 1975. In this case, too, the ozone belt is likely to be seriously upset, though at a slower rate. A crucial problem in this process is illustrated by Case 3 : that of ecological time-lag. Even if the release of chlorofluorocarbons can be checked completely today, the decomposition of ozone by the waste gases released previously will still rise until 1990, and only then will it decline slowly over the years. The results indicated are based on the most optimistic assumptions. The American scientists point out that the reality could be considerably worse, since in their calculations for the chlorofluorocarbon molecule (CF_2Cl_2 and $CFCl_3$) they have taken account of the release and catalytic effect of only one chlorine atom in each case. It is highly probable, nonetheless, that all four halogen atoms (and therefore the fluorine atoms as well) per molecule will display the effects described.

Ozone

Ozone develops as a result of photochemical processes at altitudes of over 30 km (19 miles). Molecular oxygen (O_2) separates into two oxygen atoms under the effects of ultraviolet sunlight (with a wavelength of 240 nanometers). An oxygen atom formed in this way can combine with an oxygen molecule (O_2) to form a triatomic oxygen molecule (O_3 or ozone). The O_3 molecule, for its part, rapidly absorbs ultraviolet light in the region of a wavelength of 300 nm and again separates into O_2 molecules and oxygen atoms.

Some of the oxygen atoms combine again with O_2 molecules. In this way a photochemical balance is established. Other gases also participate in these processes by purely chemical reactions. The ozone that is formed at altitudes of over 30 km finds its way into lower levels of the atmosphere only as a result of air turbulence. For this reason, the high O_3 concentrations are found in the atmosphere at altitudes of between 20 and 30 km (12 and 19 miles), while in the layer of air close to the earth only very low proportions are recorded. Enrichment of the ozone in lower air layers is not possible, since on coming into contact with the organic substances of firm ground, or with the sharply articulated upper surfaces of woodlands, ozone gives off the third oxygen atom to the organic substances and so returns to the state of molecular oxygen. The atmosphere of big cities are polluted by nitric oxide and other noxious gases, a reaction between ultraviolet radiation and these noxious gases can result in the formation of ozone.

The nitrogen dioxide contained in vehicle exhaust fumes, for instance, decomposes under solar radiation through photodissociation into nitrogen monoxide and atomic oxygen. Atomic oxygen combines with molecular oxygen, as already described, to form ozone. This explains why, in a smog situation in the daytime, the O_3 concentration in the air layer close to the ground in big cities can rise to five times the normal content and in extreme cases to a thousand times the normal content.

Ozone can cause irritation of the respiratory passages. It penetrates much deeper into the lungs than sulfur oxide. At very high concentrations the surfaces of the respiratory tract are so seriously affected that lethal pulmonary edema may result. Experiments with animals have shown, however, that repeated inhalations of ozone at low concentrations can promote a certain resistance to its irritant effects. Animals that were exposed for a long time to low concentrations of ozone did not die when exposed to higher generally fatal concentrations. It was also found that in animals that were exposed for months to near-lethal doses of ozone a thickening of the bronchiole walls occurred, as in the early stages of chronic bronchitis in human beings. Whether ultimately there is any connection between the ozone concentration in industrial agglomerations and the frequency of chronic bronchial complaints has not been established.

Human activities may affect the balance among the processes controlling ozone concentrations in the stratosphere, when chemicals emitted by cultural processes reach it. Most impacts affect ozone consumption and lead to a depletion of stratospheric ozone. Four sources of chemicals that may deplete ozone are recognized: fertilizers, high-flying aircraft, release of chlorinated compounds, and nuclear weapons.

Nitrogen-containing compounds may be released during the manufacture and consumption of industrial fertilizer for agriculture. The production and consumption of fertilizers release nitrous oxide (N_2O) which can be chemically converted to nitrogen dioxide and, after circulation to the stratosphere, added to the concentration of nitrogen compounds consuming ozone. The high concentrations of nitrous oxide released to the troposphere by natural processes are responsible for the very low conentrations of ozone in the troposphere. Unfortunately, however, the reactions controlling nitrous-oxide release from the earth by human activities are not sufficiently well known to allow quantitative evaluations of how much to get to the stratosphere.

Nitrogen and hydrogen molecules may be released in the stratosphere from jet engine exhaust. Supersonic aircraft, which fly faster and at higher altitudes than subsonic aircraft, produce the greater quantities of these compounds. In the early 1970s substantial controversy arose over the environmental effects of developing supersonic commercial aircraft (SSTs). Model calculations conducted at the time suggested that a hypothetical fleet of five hundred SSTs could release enough nitrogen compounds to deplete the ozone layer of earth by 8 to 14 percent. They also showed that a small fleet of SSTs, of the type flying in the 1970s, would have no detectable effect on stratospheric ozone. Recent discoveries concerning the chemistry of the compounds released by the SSTs suggest that effects on the ozone layer might be less than originally estimated.

A number of the gases synthesized for use by modern society and released to the atmosphere contain chlorine groups attached to organic molecules. Because some of those compounds do not readily participate in chemical reactions (they are inert) they do not break down in the troposphere. Once they diffuse to the stratosphere, where radiant energy is very intense, these inert compounds may be ionized.

Ionization of chlorinated compounds in the stratosphere releases free chlorine (Cl), which consumes ozone by the formation of chlorine oxide (ClO) and by speeding up the reaction of nitrogen oxides with ozone. The synthetic chlorinated compounds that reach the stratosphere in the greatest abundance are the chlorofluorocarbons, also known as chlorofluoromethanes (CFMs, or freons). The most abundant of the chlorofluoromethanes are trichlorofluoromethane (CCl_3F) and dichlorodifluoromethane (CCL_2F_2).

Chlorofluo-romethanes are extremely versatile chemicals. They are used as propellants in spray cans and as coolants in refrigerators, freezers, air conditioners, and the fast-freezing processing of foods; as solvents for cleaning garments and electronic components and for sterilizing medical equipment. They also are employed to blow polystyrene and polyurethane foams into place in applications such as insulations, seat cushions, and fabric backings. Because their chemical inertness (the same quality that allows them to be transported to the stratosphere) is very useful, new applications for chlorofluoromethanes continue to be found.

The reactions by which chlorofluoromethanes are ionized and consume ozone in the stratosphere were first discovered in 1979 in laboratory experiments. Subsequent research has demonstrated the efficiencies of most of the reactions involved in the complex chemistry of chlorofluoromethanes in the stratosphere. Mathematical models have been developed to describe those reactions. Most chemists hypothesize that the models depict the chemical reactions of chlorofluoromethanes in the stratosphere with reasonable accuracy. The transport of chemicals from the surface of the earth to the stratosphere occurs slowly, as does the ionization of chlorofluoromethane, and the subsequent ozone consumption. If chlorofluoromethanes are discharged at a constant rate, fifty years will pass before their full effects are felt. From the original calculations in 1974, it was estimated that the rate of chlorofluoromethane release in 1975, if held constant would deplete stratospheric ozone by 7 percent in fifty years. Continued experimentation more recently showed that some of the reactions involved in ozone depletion were more consumptive than originally estimated.

Moreover, chlorofluoromethane release rates continued to grow through the 1970s. More recent estimates from model calculations indicate that a continuation of chlorofluoromethane release for fifty years at the 1977 rate of release would deplete ozone concentrations in the stratosphere by approximately 16 percent. If world production of chlorofluoromethane continues to grow at an annual rate of 7 per cent between 1980 and 2000, as projected by some studieds, the depletion of ozone eventually could reach 30 per cent.

The high temperatures in a nuclear fireball produce nitrogen oxides in the atmosphere by combining nitrogen and oxygen. The nuclear blast carries the nitrogen oxides to the stratosphere. Once in the stratosphere nitrogen oxides consume ozone. Thus a sufficiently large nuclear war could have a global impact on human life and ecosystems far beyond the already incomprehensible impacts of the explosions and the spread of radiation, by consuming the ozone shield that protects all life on earth.

The ozone layer of the stratosphere reduces the total radiant energy penetrating to earth by only 2 per cent. Like most chemicals, however, ozone absorbs some wave-lengths of energy more efficiently than it does others. Concentrations of .ozone in the stratosphere are sufficient to remove more than 95 percent of the radiant energy with wavelength between 290 and 320 nanometers. These wavelengths are called ultraviolet-B (UV-B) or damaging ultraviolet (DUV) radiation. Most complex forms of life on earth have evolved since the ozone layer was established—in an environment almost free of UV-B radiation.

Most life forms tend to be especially sensitive to increases in UV-B radiation. Mathematical models estimate that a 16 per cent reduction in stratospheric ozone would increase UV-B penetration to the earth by 40 per cent and a 30 per cent reduction in ozone would double UB-B penetration. The most important human health impact from increasing UV-B radiation would be inducing skin cancer. Two general types of skin cancer are melanoma and nonmelanoma. Nonmelanoma is the most common form. Its incidence is estimated at 300,000 to 600, 000 cases per year in the United States. Nonmelanoma skin cancers are rarely fatal and can usually be removed surgically.

Melanoma is a more severe cancer that is fatal approximately one third of the time. Both types of skin cancer increase with increased exposure to UV-B radiation. Incidence of both increase from high latitudes toward the equator, as the intensity of radiant energy (and UV-B) penetration increases. Similarly, skin cancer incidences increase with increased voluntary exposure to sunlihgt. In 1980 a National Academy of Sciences panel report on the effects of ozone depletion concluded that the 16 per cent reduction in stratospheric ozone projected from chloro-fluoromethane discharge "would lead to a certainty of very many thousands of additional cases every year of nonmelanoma skin cancer and a likely probability of thousands of new cases per year of melanoma of which a substantial fraction would be fatal". Other impacts from ozone depletion also are possible. Twenty per cent of one hundred varieties of agricultural crops were found to give reduced yields at slightly increased doses of UV-B radiation, when tested in the laboratory.

Sensitivities were less evident in some of the varieties in tests in actual agricultural plots. At least some crops (sugar beets, tomatoes, corn, and mustard) might suffer reduced yields if penetration of UV-B radiation is increased. Changes in UV-B penetration on the ecosystems of the earth are also possible. Small aquatic organisms are sensitive to increased levels of UV-B radiation, but they may be protected by absorption of the radiation by the water. Like humans, other life forms on earth are adapted to life at low levels of UV-B radiation. Simplification of biological communities occurs when they are exposed to low levels of gamma radiation, suggesting that species extictions could occur through a global increase in radiation exposures.

Major controversy exists concerning the effects on ozone in the stratosphere of human releases of nitrogen and chlorine compounds. The main source of the controversy is the accuracy of the models involved in calculating the effects. The models have been developed purely from laboratory experiments, which may oversimplify the complexities of interactions occurring in the stratosphere. Confirmation of the model projections depends on measuring a decline in ozone concentrations as pollutant concentrations increase. The difficulties in obtaining information from the stratosphere, and the natural variability of ozone in the stratosphere, limit the accuracy of measuring an ozone decline. A 4 to 5 per cent reduction in ozone must occur before chemists can be sure a decline is in progress (Maugh 1979). Depletion resulting from chlorofluoromethane, up to 1980, is estimated from the models to be 2 per cent—below the level of detection.

A detectable 5 per cent depletion of ozone is not expected until 2000. Until an actual depletion is measured, verification of the laboratory evidence will not be possible. If all production of chlorofluoromethane were stopped upon observance of a 5 percent reduction in 2000, the total ozone depletion would be 7 per cent, as chlorofluoromethane released prior to 2000 migrated to the stratosphere. Any delay in stopping releases would magnify the extent of the problem in the future. The photochemical reactions that deplete ozone have been convincingly demonstrated in laboratory experiments.

Most atmospheric chemists believe that those reactions projects effects on ozone with reasonable accuracy. Other chemists, however, suggest that the role of photochemical reactions in controlling ozone in the stratosphere may be less than projected from the models. These workers argue that in several types of situations (nuclear bomb tests and variations in ozone with variations inputs of ionizing radiant energy), measurements of changes in ozone in the stratosphere do not agree with model projections.

Chemical reactions in the stratosphere itself may not be as important in controlling ozone as such processes as the transport of gases between the troposphere and the stratosphere. These arguments do not disprove the ozone models, but they do emphasize that some uncertainty will plague the projections until the atmosphere itself performs enough of the experiment for the results to be detectable. In the late 1970s, the use of chlorofluoromethane as a propellant in most spray cans was banned in the United States. This move reduced chlorofluoromethane discharge rates back to levels characteristic of before 1973. The economic impact was small. Regulation of chlorofluoromethane release has not occurred outside the United States and its use is increasing else-where. The fluorochemical industry suggests that more research is essential before regulation of chlorofluoromethane is imposed.

The scientists who have prepared reports on the subject for the National Academy of Sciences consider that the laboratory studies provide convincing evidence that the "hypothesis" of an effect is correct, and that further delay in regulating chlorofluormethane release will only increase the eventual problem. If the release of nitrous oxide from agricultural fertilizers is shown to also effect ozone concentrations, then regulation of chlorofluoromethane will become an even more significant issue. The effect of a growth in both nitrous oxide and chlorofluoromethane releases on ozone might be to encourage much faster depletion rates than projected at present. (Nitrous oxide is not included in present projections because controls on its release are not sufficiently understood). Cutbacks in fertilizer consumption are not realistic, given the world demand for food. Regulation of chlorofluoromethane discharge might then become essential if human impacts on the radiation shield of the biosphere are to be minimized.

Particulates

Small solid particles and liquid droplets, collectively called particulates, are present in the air in great numbers, and at times they constitute a serious pollution problem. Many different chemical substances can enter the atmosphere in particulate form. The wide range in chemical composition of products from a single source, coal combustion, is shown in Table 1.

Table 1

Fly Ash Composition (Coal Combustion)

Component (% Calculated As)	*Percentage of Fly Ash*
Carbon	0.37-36.2
Iron (as Fe_2O_3 or Fe_3O_4	2.0-26.8
Magnesium (as MgO)	0.06-4.77
Calcium (as CaO)	0.12-14.73
Aluminium (as Al_2O_3)	9.81-58.4
Sulfur (as SO_2)	0.12-24.33
Titanium (as TiO_2)	0-2.8
Carbonate (as CO_3^-)	0-2.6
Silicon (as SiO_2)	17.3-63.6
Phosphorus (as P_2O_2)	0.07-47.2
Potassium (as K_2O)	2.8-3 0
Sodium (as Na_2O)	0.2-09
Undetermined	0.08-18.9

Due to the large variety substances encountered, a general discussion of chemical properties cannot be made for particulate pollutants.

Many physical properties may apply to particulates in general. The most important of these is size, which ranges from a diameter of 0.0002 μ (about the size of a small molecule) to a diameter of about 500 μ. The micron (μh) is a commonly used unit in particulate pollution work and is equal to 10^{-6} metres. In the size ranges given above, particles are having lifetime in the suspended state of something between a few seconds and several months. This lifetime depends upon the settling rate, which in turn depends upon the size and density of the particles and the turbulence of the air.

A second property of particulates is their ability to act as sites for sorption. This property has been a function of surface area, which is large for most particulates. The process of sorption occurs when an individual molecule impacts on the surface of a particulate and does not rebound, but sticks or sorbs. Obviously the optical properties of particles are exerting an important effect upon air quality. Particles less than approximately 0.1μ in diameter scatter light much like molecules, i.e., Rayleigh scattering. Generally, such small particles are exerting an in significant effect upon visibility in the atmosphere.

The light scattering and intercepting properties of particles larger than 1μ are almost proportional to the particle cross-sectional area. Particles having diameters between 0.1μ and 1μ are of sizes having the same order of magnitude as the wavelengths of visible light. The optical properties are important in the determination of effects of atmospheric particulates on solar radiation and visibility. Very small solid particles are carbon black, silver iodide, combustion nuclei, and sea salt nuclei. Larger particles are cement dust, windblown soil dust, foundry dust, and pulverized coal.

Liquid particulate matter, generally categorized as "mist", includes rain drops, fog, and sulfuric acid mist. Some particulate matter is biological material, such as very small viruses, bacteria, bacterial spores, fungal spores, and pollen. Particulate matter may be organic or inorganic; both types have been very important atmospheric contaminants.

Particulate matter originates through a wide variety of processes which are ranging from simple grinding of bulk matter to complicated chemical or biochemical syntheses. The effects of particulate matter are also widely varied. Either by itself, or in combination with gaseous pollutants, particulate matter may be detrimental to human health. Atmospheric particles are able to damage materials reduce visibility, and bring about undesirable esthetic effects.

The units used to express concentrations of particulates are micrograms per cubic metre of air (μg/m). In order to convert from μg/m^3 to ppm on a volume basis, the molecular weight of the particulate is needed. No acceptable particulates molecular weights are available because of the diverse composition of particulates. The number of particles in the atmosphere have been found to vary from several hundred per cubic centimetre in ultra clean air to more than 100,000 per cubic centimeter in highly polluted atmospheres.

Most of the particulate mass in the atmosphere occurs in the size range of 0.1 μ to 10 μ. In remote areas the levels of atmospheric particulate mass may be as low as 10 μg/m^3. In urban areas average levels of 60 μg/m^3 to 220 μg/m^3 are generally encountered, and levels may range up to the vicinity of 2000 μg/m^3. The size and composition of particulate matter have been found to vary diurnally and with weather conditions. Furthermore, the elemental composition differs markedly with particle size, and this may exert a strong influence upon the toxicological effects of particulate matter. For example, calcium tends to occur in large particles which are produced from wind erosion of soil, rock quarrie's cement, and similar sources.

Likewise, the common soil components—iron, manganese, potassium and titanium—generally occur in large particles. Lead and bromine occur to a large extent in smaller particles, around the 0.5 μ size. A particular toxicological hazard is presented, because particles in the range of 0.015-1 μ have been most efficiently retained in the respiratory system. These two elements are found together in atmospheric particulate matter and get produced to a large extent by automobile exhausts.

Numerous natural processes release particulate matter into the atmosphere. Typical of these processes are volcano eruptions and the blowing of dust and soil by the wind. The activities of man also release; for example, in the form of dust and absestos particulates from construction, fly ash from smelters and mining operations, and smoke from incomplete combustion processes.

The particles above approximately 1m in size are formed by the disintegration of larger particles. This is a dispersion process, and the product is termed as a dispersion aerosol. Dusts are solid dispersion aerosols. Many dispersion aerosols originate from natural sources. Sea spray, windblown dust, and volcanic dust of course preceded man. Cultivation of land has made it much easier for the wind to pick up topsoil and blow it over great distances.

Much are more energy is needed to break material down into small particles than is needed (or released) to synthesize particles, through adhesion of smaller particles or through chemical processes. That is the reason that most dispersion particles are relatively large. These larger particles in general having fewer harmful effects than do very small particles.

Chemical Processes for Particle Formaiton

Metal oxides form a major class of inorganic particles in the atmosphere. These are produced whenever fuels containing metals are burned. For example, during the combustion of pyrite-containing coal,

$$3FeS_2 + 8O_2 \rightarrow Fe_3O_4 + 6SO_2 \quad \ldots(1)$$

particulate iron oxide is formed. Organic vanadium in residual fuel oil gets converted to particulate vanadium oxide. Part of the calcium carbonate in the ash fraction of coal gets converted to calcium oxide,

$$CaCO_3 + \text{heat} \rightarrow CaO + CO_2 \quad ..(2)$$

and goes to the atmosphere through the stack.

A special case of particulate matter formed during the combustion of fuel is that of the particulate lead halides which are formed in the burning of leaded gasoline. Tetraethyl lead in leaded gasoline reacts with oxygen and halogenated scavengers,

$$Pb(C_2H_4)_4 + O_2 + \text{halogenated} \rightarrow \text{scavengers}$$

$$CO_2 + H_2O + PbCl_2 + PbBrCl + PbBr_2 \quad ...(3)$$

to form lead halides which are volatile enough to exit through the exhaust system, but which condense to form particles. By this pathway some lead has been entering the atmosphere.

A common process for the formation of aerosol mists involves the oxidation of atmospheric sulfur dioxide to sulfuric acid,

$$2SO_2 + O_2 + 2H_2O \rightarrow 2H_2SO_4 \quad ...(4)$$

a hygroscopic substance which accumulates atmospheric water to form small liquid droplets. In the presence of basic air pollutants, such as ammonia or calcium oxide, the sulfuric acid reacts to form salts:

$$H_2SO_4 \text{ (droplet)} + 2NH_3\text{(gas)} = (NH_4)_2SO_4\text{(droplet)} ...(5)$$

$$H_2SO_4\text{(droplet)} + CaO\text{(particle)} = CaSO_4\text{(droplet)} + H_2O. \quad ...(6)$$

Under conditions of low humidity water gets lost from these droplets and a solid aerosol is formed.

The three most important surface properties of particles include nucleation, adhesion, and sorption. Nucleation is involved in raindrop formation. Adhesion, or coagulation, refers to the process by which extremely small particles form larger aggregates and eventually reach a size at which they settle rapidly. Liquid particles of the same composition are very likely to adhere to one another when they collide. The likelihood of solid particles adhering to one another tend to increase with decreasing particle size.

Sorption designates the phenomenon by which molecules are taken up particles. If the vapour or gas is dissolved within the particle, the phenomenon is termed as absorption. Adsorption refers to sorption on the surface of the particle. Chemisorption refers to sorption involving a specific chemical interaction like the reaction of atmospheric CO_2 with particles of $Ca(OH)_2$:

$$Ca(OH)_2 + CO_2 \rightarrow CaCO_3 + H_2O$$

Other examples of chemisorption include the reactions of sulfur dioxide with aluminium oxide or iron oxide aerosols and the reaction of sulfuric acid aerosols and ammonia.

The proportions of elements in atmospheric particulate matter reflect the relative abundances of elements in the parent material. This provides a good idea of the source of much particulate matter. For example, particulate matter largely from ocean spray origin in a coastal area receiving sulfur dioxide pollution may show anomalously high sulfate and correspondingly low chloride. The sulfate comes from atmospheric oxidation of sulfur dioxide to form nonvolatile ionic sulfate, whereas some chloride may get lost from the solid aerosol as volatile HCl.

$$2SO_2 + O_2 + 2H_2O = 2H_2SO_4 \quad ...(1)$$

$$H_2SO_4 = 2NaCl \text{ (particulate)} = Na_2SO_4 \text{ (particulate)} + 2HCl \text{ (gas)} \quad ...(2)$$

Atmospheric particulate matter is having an extremely wide diversity of chemical composition. Organic matter, nitrogen compounds, sulfur compounds, a number of metals, and radionuclides occur in the particulate matter in polluted urban atmospheres.

An extensive analysis of particulate matter collected from a large number of sampling stations in urban locations showed the following composition of particulate matter in units of μg/m^3 (arithmetic averages of biweekly samples): total suspended particulates (105), ammonium (1.3), nitrate (2.6), sulfate (10.6), benzene-soluble organics (6.8), antimony (0.01), arsenic (0.02), cadmium (0.002), chromium (0.015), copper (0.09), iron (1.58), lead (0.79), manganese (0.10), nikel (0.034), tin (0.02), titanium (0.04), vanadium (0.050), and zinc (0.67). Molybdenum occurred at an average level of > 0.005 μg/m^3 although a maximum value of 0.78 μg/m was observed.

The average levels of beryllium, bismuth, and cobalt found were all less than 0.0005 μg/m^3 although maximum values of 0.010, 0.064, and 0.060 μ/m^3, respectively, were observed. Although it is not included in the above list, sodium is a common element found in particulate matter in coastal areas. Sodium enters the atmosphere as sodium chloride in sea spray aerosol particles. Levels of approximately 1 μg/m^3 of sodium are not uncommon in coastal areas. Radionuclides occurred in the particulate matter, with a gross beta radio activity of 0.8 pico Curies/m^3, and a maximum value of 12.4 pCi/m^3. At various times of the year or day and in different locations any of the trace elements which are of concern for their toxicological effects are found in atmospheric particles. Table 2 shows some elements found in particulate matter collected at Tucoson, Arizona.

Table 2

Trace Elements from a Typical Particulate Sample

Element	*Concentration* µg/m³ of air	*Element*	*Concentration* µg/m³ of air
Al	4.1	Li	0.003
Be	0.00003	Mg	1.3
Bi	0.003	Mn	0.012
Ca	10.4	Na	2.2
Cd	0.020	Ni	0.013
Co	0.0015	Pb	0.8
Cr	0.004	Rb	0.003
Cs	0.0004	Si	13.4
Cu	0.6	Sr	0.022
Fe	3.3	Ti	0.15
K	2.8	V	0.009
		Zn	0.14

Some of the metals found in polluted atmospheres are hazardous to human health. All except beryllium belong to the classification of heavy metals. Some idea of the relative dangers of these metals may be gained from the values allowed in atmospheres to which healthy industrial workers are allowed exposure during an eight-hour day. The value for each metal is known as a threshold limit value, TLV. The TLVs of metals have been compared with their concentrations in a number of urban air samples. The results are summarized in Table 3.

Mercury in the atmosphere has been a cause of great concern due to its toxicity. Elemental mercury is volatile, and much of the mercury entering the atmosphere does so in atomic form. Most of the mercury entering the atmosphere from coal combustion and volcanoes does so as the elemental form.

Table 3

Toxic Metals in the Atmosphere Compared to TLV and Average Levels Found in Urban Atmospheres.

Metal (descending order of toxicity	*TLV mg/m³ (range denotes different toxic forms)*	*Average metal level: TLV*
Be	0.002	less than 0.00025
Hg	0.01—0.05	0.002
Cd	0.1	0.0001
Pb	0.1—0.2	0.004
As	0.2—0.5	0.00004
V	0.5	0.0002
Ni	0.007—1.0	0.00003
Cu	1.0	0.00009
Fe	1.0	0.0003
Zn	1.0	0.0001

Some mercury in the atmosphere gets associated with particulate matter. Volatile organomercury compounds such as dimethylmercury, $(CH_3)_2Hg$, also occur in the atmosphere. Monomethylmercury salts, such as $(CH_3)HgBr$, are also volatile mercury compounds which sometimes occur in the atmosphere. Most coals are having appreciable levels of mercury, and this presents a problem which must be dealt with as the use of coal inevitably increases.

Lead is probably the most serious atmospheric heavy metal pollutant. Deecreasing use of leaded gasoline and increasing use of coal will probably result in its replacement by mercury as the most troublesome atmospheric metal. The lead halides from automotive exhausts are the most common form of atmospheric lead. Of these, lead bromochloride PbBrCl, predominates. Appreciable amounts of $NH_4Cl.2PbBrCl$, and ammonium chloride-lead bromochloride double salt, also occur in auto exhausts. The atmospheric reactions and ultimate fate of this lead are subject to conflicting opinions.

Beryllium in the Atmosphere

Beryllium is used primarily as a component of specially alloys. Some of the primary uses include electrical equipment, electronic instrumentation, space gear, and nuclear equipment. Its distribution is by no means comparable to that of other toxic metals such as lead or mercury. Because of its specialty uses, however, consumption of beryllium is increasing. Beryllium has the lowest allowable TLV of any metal, and its presence in the atmosphere is very hazardous.

Asbestos in the Atmosphere

Asbestos is a naturally-occurring fibrous silicate. The fibers are separable, yielding fine filaments. Small fibers of asbestos irritate lung tissue causing a condition called "asbestosis". This condition is characterized by lung fibrosis. Therefore, atmospheric asbestos is a matter of considerable concern.

Mineral Particulate Matter from Combustion—Fly Ash

Much of the mineral Particulate matter in a polluted atmosphere is in the form of oxides and other compounds produced during the combustion of high-ash fossil fuel. Most of the mineral matter in fossil fuels such as coal or lignite is converted during combustion to a fused, glassy bottom ash which presents no air pollution problems. Smaller ash particles called fly ash enter urnace flues and, in a properly equipped stack system, are collected efficiently. However, a certain percentage of this fly ash escapes through the stack and enters the atmosphere. Unfortunately, these tend to be the smaller particles which do the most damage to human health, plants, and visibility.

Radionuclides in the Atmosphere

A significant natural source of radionuclides in the atmosphere is the noble gas radon, product of the decay of radium. Radon may enter the atmosphere as one of two isotopes. ^{222}Rn and ^{220}Rn. Both are alpha emitters with half-lives of 3.8 days and 54.5 seconds, respectively. Also, cosmic rays act on nuclei in the atmosphere to produce radionuclides including ^{7}Be, ^{10}Be, ^{14}C, ^{39}Cl, ^{3}H, ^{22}Na, ^{32}P and ^{33}P. One of the more serious problems in connection with radon appears to be that of radioactivity originating from uranium mill tailings.

Some medical authorities have postulated that the rate of birth defects and infant cancer in areas where uranium mill tailings have been employed in residential construction are significantly higher than normal. The combustion of fossil fuels introduces radoactivity into the atmosphere in the form of radionuclides contained in fly ash. Large coalfired power plants lacking ash control equipment may introduce up to several hundred milicicuries of radionuclides into the atmosphere each year.

The radioactive noble gas ^{35}Kr goes into the atmosphere by the operation of nuclear reactors and the processing of spent reactor fuels. The detonation of nuclear weapons above ground contributes a great deal to particulate radioactive material. Such material may be carried through the atmosphere for tremendous distances, eventually to be scavenged from the atmosphere by rain. For example, about a week after a nuclear detonation in China on December 24, 1967, the following radionuclides were found in rain in Fayetteville, Arkansas: ^{91}Y, ^{141}Ce, ^{144}Ce, ^{147}Nd, ^{147}Pm, ^{149}Pm ^{151}Sm, ^{153}Sm, ^{155}Eu, ^{89}Sr, ^{90}Sr, ^{115m}Cd, ^{129m}Te, ^{131}I, ^{132}Te, ^{140}Ba. The rate of travel of radioactive particle through the atmosphere is a function of particle size. Appreciables fractionation of nuclear debris is observed because of the difference in rate of transport.

Organic Particulate Matter

Organic particulate matter is found in a wide variety of compounds in the atmosphere. It is interesting to note that a so called "average formula" of this organic matter, collected from 200 U.S. areas and isolated as a benzene-extractable fraction, is $C_{32.4}H_{48}O_{3.8}S_{0.083}$ (hologen)$_{0.065}$ (alkoxy)$_{0.12}$. Much of this organic matter occurs in the respirable 1μ size range. The aliphatic fraction of the neutral group is having a high percentage of long-chain hydrocarbons, predominantly those containing from 16 to 28 carbon atoms. Such hydrocarbons are not though to be particularly significant health hazard, or to participate strongly in atmospheric chemistry reactions.

Many of the hydrocarbons found in the aromatic fraction, however, are polynuclear aromatics, and some are proven carcinogens (cancer-causing agents). Therefore, these hydrocarbons are particularly important as air pollutants. Aldehydes, ketones, epoxides, esters, quinones, and lactones are found among the oxygenated neutral organic components. A few of these compounds may be mutagenic or carcinogenic. The acidic fractions are having long-chain fatty acids and nonvolatile phpenols. Among the acids recovered from air pollutant particulate matter are lauric, myristic, palmitic, stearic, behenic, oleic, and linoleic. The basic fraction consists largely of alkaline N-heterocyclic hydrocarbons, such as acridine.

At the present time comparatively little is known about the chemical constitution and environmental significance of the basic fraction. A significant portion of organic particulate matter coming from automotive exhausts has been characterized as "oxidized, polymerized hydrocarbons and nitrogenous azaheterocyclic substances".

Table 4

Types of Organic Compounds Found in Respirable Organic Matter along Highways.

Type of compound	*Possible effect*
Polar organics	Extracted by aqueous body fluids enabling penetration of tissue in a soluble form.
Aldehydes	Suspected of being the primary causative agents in smoke poisoning, postulated denaturation of amino acids and RNA. This causes inflamation and necrosis of tissue.
Other oxygenated organics (acids, neutral oxygen compounds)	Some have suspected carcino genic effects.
Polynuclear azahetero cyclinc compounds (benza cridines, dibenzacridines, benzoquinolones)	Some of these, such as dibenz (a, h)-acridine and dibenz (a, j) acridine are known carcinogens.

Relatively little research has been done on the effects of particulate pollution on vegetation. Most of what has been done has been concerned with specific dusts rather than the conglomerate mixture usually present in the atmosphere. This dust, when combined with a mist or light rain, formed a thick crust on upper leaf-surfaces which was found to interfere with photosynthesis in the plant by shielding out needed sunlight and upsetting the process of CO_2 exchange with the atmosphere. The growth of such plants was inhibited. A possible indirect effect of particulates deposited on plants is the chance that the particulates might contain chemical components harmful to animals that use the plants as food.

The only major route by which particles enter the body through the respiratory tract. Relatively large particles are likely to get retained in the nasal cavity and in the pharynx. Very small particles are likely to reach the lungs and to be retained by them. The respiratory system is having mechanisms for the removal of particulate matter. In the ciliated region, particles are carried as far as the entrance to the gastrointestinal tract by a flow of mucus. Macrophages in the nonciliated pulmonary regions carry particles to the ciliated region. The respiratory system may get damaged directly by particulate material. It may enter the blood system or lymph system through the lungs.

In addition, the particulate material or soluble components of it may get transported to organs some distance from the lungs and have a detrimental effect on these organs. Particles cleared from the respiratory tract largely enter the gastrointestinal tract. Material may also enter the blood after it is transported to the gastrointestinal tract. A strong correlation exists between the daily mortality rate and acute episodes of air pollution. In such cases, high levels of particulate matter are accompanied by high levels of SO_2 and other pollutants.

Particles over 5.0 μ in diameter are stopped and deposited mainly in the nose and the throat. Those that do penetrate to the lungs do not often go beyond the air ducts or bronchi, and even these are soon removed by ciliary action. Particles ranging in size from 0.5—5.0 μ in diameter can be deposited in lung as far as the bronchioles. Few reach the alveoli. Most particles deposited in the bronchioles are removed by the cilia within the two hours. Particles less than 0.5 in diameter reach and may settle in the alveoli. The removal of such particles from these areas is much less rapid and less complete than from the larger passages. Some of the particles retained in the alveoli are absorbed into the blood. Particulate matter which enters and remains in the lungs can exert a toxic effect in three different ways.

1. The particles may be intrinsically toxic because of chemical or physical characteristics. More will be said later about this type of particle.
2. The particles may be inert themselves but once in the respiratory tract they may interfere with the removal of other more harmful material.
3. The particles may carry adsorbed or absorbed irritating gas molecules and thus enable such molecules to reach and remain in sensitive areas of the lungs. Carbon, in the form of soot, is a common particulate with a very good ability to sorb gas molecules on the surface.

Intrinsically toxic particulates are not commonly found in the atmosphere in high concentrations except for sulfuric acid aerosol. However, many toxic particles are found in the air in trace amounts. Table 5. contains information about a number of trace metals in this category that may pose health hazards in the environment.

Table 5

Trace Metals that may pose Health Hazards in the Environment

Element	*Sources*	*Health Effects*
Nickel	Diesel oil, residual oil, coal, tobacco smoke, chemicals and catalysts, steel and nonferrous alloys	Lung cancer (as carbonyl)

Beryllium	Coal, industry (new uses proporsed in nuclear power industry, as rocket fuel)	Acute and chronic syste poison, cancer
Boron	Coal, cleaning agents, medicinals, glass making, other industrial	Nontoxic except as borane
Germanium	Coal	Little innate toxicity
Arsenic	Coal, petroleum, detergents, pesticides, mine tailings	Hazard disputed, may cause cancer
Selenium	Coal, sulfur	May cause dental caries, carcinogenic in rats, essential to mammals in low doses
Yttrium	Coal, petroleum	Carcinogenic in mice over lon-term exposure
Mercury	Coal, electrical batteries, other industrial	Nerve damage and death
Vanadium	Petroleum (Venezuela, Iran), chemicals and catalysts, steel and nonferrous alloys	Probably no hazard at current levels
Cadmium	Coal, zinc mining, water mains and pipes, tobacco smoke	Cardiovascular disease and hypertension in humans suspected interferes with zinc and copper metabolism
Antimony	Industry	Shortened life span in rats.
Lead	Auto exhaust (from gasoline), paints (prior to about 1948)	Brain damage, convulsions, behavioural disorders, death.

The poisonous nature of beryllium and its compounds has been recognized for years. Soluble compounds such as $BeSO_4$ and $BeCl_2$ commonly produce acute inflammation of the lungs. Beryllium metal or insoluble compounds cause the chronic pulmonary disease, berylliosis. Coal burning is another source of atmospheric beryllium because most coal contains beryllium as an impurity. Recent findings indicate that inhalation of asbestos, a substance used for insulation by the building trade, can produce serious problems in previously healthy lungs.

Table 6

Beryllium Exposure Limits Set by the AEC

AEC Exposure Limit ($\mu g/m^3$)	Conditions	Measured Atmospheric Levels $\mu g/m^3$)	Conditions
25	Industrial limit for short-term exposure	0.028—0.083	Concentration in vicinity of a beryllium plant
2.	Industrial limit averaged an eight hour work period	0.008	Maximum ambient air value
0.01	Industrial limit averaged over 30 days for people living in the neighbourhood of a beryllium plant	0.0005	Daily average air value

Airborne particles, including soot, dust, fumes, and mist can bring about a wide range of damage to materials. The extent and type of damage have been found to depend upon the chemical composition and physical state of the pollutant. Passive damage is caused when particulates settle on and soil materials, creating a need for more frequent cleaning. The cleaning processes weaken the materials.

Chemical damage results when the particulates themselves are corrosive, or when they carry absorbed or absorbed corrosive substances along with them. Metals are generally resistant to corrosion in dry air and even in clean air that are having only small amounts of water. Particulates accelerate corrosion, especially in the presence of sulfur-containing compounds.

The ability of particulates to damage and soil buildings, sculpture, and other structures is especially more common in cites where large amounts of coal and sulfur-bearing oils are used. The resulting particulates are generally tarry, sticky, and acidic so they adhere to surfaces and behave as acid reservoirs for corrosion. Painted surfaces are very susceptible to particulate damage before the paint is dry. In addition, some particulate fumes and mists react directly with dry painted surfaces, and bring about considerable damage. This type of paint damage is common on automobiles frequently parked near industrial plants. The soiling of textile materials has been one of the most important harmful effects from particulates.

Particulates in the atmosphere are known to exert a definite influence on the amount and type of solar radiation that reaches the surface of the earth. This influence is the result of light scattering and absorption by the particulates. One principal effect is the reduction of visibility. The eye has difficulty in distinguishing between the object and the background. Decreased visibility creates obvious problems, some dangerous (aircraft or automobile operation) and some just annoying (sightseeing, and so forth).

Illumination problems are created by particulate pollution. In some cities the processes of scattering and absorption are able to reduce by one-third or more the amount of visible light reaching the earth's surface. The gloom resulting from reduced amounts of sunlight creates a heavy need for artificial illumination, which in turn require more power which could mean that more pollutants from the power plant will be released, and a cycle is created. The amount of particulate pollution tend to vary with the season. In autumn and winter, increased heating of houses, and other buildings creates a demand for mor power which causes more particulates. This perhaps accounts in part for gloomy winter day.

Particulates in the atmosphere may influence the formation of clouds, rain, and snow by acting as nuclei upon which water condensation can take place.

World-wide climate changes are also related to particulate pollution. The reduction in the amount of solar radiation reaching the earth's surface may be upsetting the delicate heat balance of the earth's atmosphere. In spite of an increase in CO_2 content of the atmosphere over the past several decades, which should cause an atmospheric temperature increase, the average world-wide temperature has been decreasing slightly since 1940s. The increased reflection of solar radiation by particulates has been more than compensating for the climatic effect of increased atmospheric CO_2.

Effect of Hydrogen Fluoride

Hydrogen fluoride behaves somewhat similar to sulphur dioxide except that with a few species of plants it is effective in causing lesions and interfering with photosynthesis in concentrations two or three orders less than in the case of sulphur dioxide. With most species it is up to 10 times as effective as sulphur dioxide. However, recovery of plants from the fluoride effect is much slower than from sulphur dioxide. This difference in rate of recovery is probably explained by the fact that sulphite in the leaves is rapidly oxidised to the relatively non-toxic sulphate, whereas fluorides can be removed only by the slower process of volatization or by some obscure chemical reaction. Forage may be rendered unsafe for animal feeding if more than 50 ppm of fluorine is absorbed.

Effect of Ozone

Ozone is phytotoxic in exposures of a few hours at about 0.2 ppm. Injury due to ozone is quite different from typical smog injury. The lesions are generally confined to the upper surface.

Fluorine

Of all farm animals, cattle and sheep are the most suceptible to fluorine toxicosis. Horses appear to be quite resistant to fluorine poisoning. Poultry are probably the most resistant to fluorine, of all farm animals.

Symptoms of Acute Fluorine Poisoning

Lack of appetite, rapid loss in weight, decline in heath and vigour, lameness, periodic diarrhoea, muscular weakness and death. Characterize the acute form of fluorine poisoning. It may also result in considerable increase of bone fluorine. But acute poisoning due to fluorides is unlikely in a majority of the cases.

Symptoms of Chronic Fluorine Poisoning

Fluorine is cumulative poison under conditions of continuous exposure to sub-acute doses. Fluorine is also a protoplasmic poison. It has a marked affinity for calcium and interferes with normal calcification. Animals have been reported to be more resistant than humans to dental mottling. Cattle and sheep are the most frequently affected animals. Teeth in the process of formation are easily affected. Hence tooth symptoms are a sensitive and unique criterion of chronic fluorosis. Excessive wearing of incisor and molar teeth may occur at high levels of fluorine intake.

Bone lesions may develop at any age. A bony overgrowth may be observed on the leg bones, jaw bones and ribs. Their appearance indicates there has been a high fluoride intake over a long period. Lameness may occur as a result of this overgrowth on the leg bones. This may be followed by stiffness of joints. Effects of fluorides on skeletal structures are usually of a permanent nature.

Symptoms of advanced fluorisis include lack of appetite, general ill-health due to malnutrition, lowered fertility, reduced milk production and growth retardation. The symptoms developed in other species such as rabbits, horses and poultry are similar to those in cattle and sheep, i.e., mottling, staining and wearing of the teeth, bony overgrowths on the skeleton, stiffiness and lethargy and general ill-health from malnutrition and starvation.

While diagnosis of chronic fluorine poisoning is done, one has to be careful. This is because drinking water supplies may contain unduly high level of fluorides. Also, mineral supplements may contribute appreciable amounts of fluorine to the diet. Hence, a check of all possible source's must be made when investigating fluorosis.

Arsenic occurs as an impurity in many ores and in coal. It has been reported to cause poisoning of livestock near various industrial processes and smelters. Just like most industrial air contaminants, arsenic may spread over a considerable area from a stack source. Arsenic in dusts or sprays on plants can lead to poisoning of cattle.

Symptoms of Acute Arsenic Poisoning

In acute cases the symptoms are severe salivation, thirst, vomiting, uneasiness, feeble and irregular pulse and respiration. The animal stamps, lies down and gets up. There is diarrhoea, and the faeces have a garlic odour and are sometimes bloody. The ears become cold, the body trembles and develops abnormal temperature and convulsion. Death may occur in few hours or days.

Symptoms of Chronic Arsenic Poisoning

Arsenic appears to have a depressing effect upon the central nervous systems. The animal becomes dull, and exhibits a lack of appetite, with a resulting weight loss. Also, there may be chronic cough and diarrhoea may occur continuously. There may be thickening of the skin, anaemia and abortion or sterlity. Chronic poisoning can result in eventual paralysis and death.

Tolerance Limits

Arsenic as well as its soluble compounds are extremely poisonous. It has been reported that sheep have been poisoned by as little as 0.25-0.50 g of arsenic daily, whereas cattle and horses may tolerate 1.3-1.9 g daily. It has also been reported from laboratory experiments, that 10 mg of arsenic per kilogram of body weight per day has produced chronic arsenic poisoning in guinea pigs. A detailed investigation of the effects of arsenic poisoning on farm animals is necessary to establish standard tolerance limits.

Symptoms of Acute Lead Poisoning

In case of acute lead poisoning the onset is sudden and the course relatively short. Prostration, staggering and inability to rise are prominent symptoms. The pulse is always fast but weak. Some animals may fall suddenly, stiffen the legs and have convulsions. There is complete loss of appetite, paralysis of the digestive tract and diarrhoea. Other nervous symptoms in cattle are grinding of the teeth and rapid chewing of the cud. In case of horse, it may result in complete loss of appetite, nervous depression, lethargy and death.

Symptoms of Chronic Lead Poisoning

Chronic lead poisoning has been observed frequently in horses that have been grazing an forage near smelters, lead mines, and in orchards that have been sprayed. Paralysis of the muscles of the larynx and difficulty in breathing are the main symptoms. Convulsions may occur from the paralysis of the throat, and the difficulty in breathing may be unusually severe and persistent, during and after exercise.

Tolerance Limits

Lead is a cumulative poison. Therefore, the continuous ingestion of even very small daily doses will be finally as effective as one toixc dose. Hence in case of slight contamination death can occur after many months and in case of severe contamination death can occur within 24 hours.

It has also been reported that inadequate calcium in diet increases the retention of lead in the animal body. Low calcium diets may result in lead storage of as much as five times as compared to that found in animals that receive sufficient amounts of calcium. However, extra quantities of calcium above the amount considered sufficient, will not offer additional protection against poisoning.

Hydrogen Sulphide and Mercaptans

Hydrogen sulphide is a foul smelling gas. It is well known for its rotten egg like odour. Exposures to hydrogen sulphide for short periods can result in fatigue of the sense of smell.

Other sulphur compounds that are of interest in air pollution mainly because of their strong odours are methyl mercaptan (CH_3SH) and ethyl mercaptan (C_2H_3SH). But it has been reported that at the concentrations at which they are odour nuisances, they have no other effect on human health. In fact, mercaptans are often added to natural or manufactured gas supplies so that leakage of gas will be noticed.

Fluorides

Fluorides present in air, range from those which are extremely irritant and corrosive like hydrogen fluoride to relatively non-reactive compounds. But fluorine is a cumulative poison even under condition of prolonged exposure and in subacute concentrations.

Lead

The main source of lead in urban atmospheres is the automobile. It creates urban concentration of inorganic lead of about 103 $\mu g/m^3$, with high values in areas of heavy traffic. Inorganic lead acts as an agent which causes a variety of human health disorders. The effects include gastro-intestinal damage, liver and kidney damage, abnormalities in fertility and pregnancy, and mental development of children gets affected.

Hydrogen Vapours

Some of the hydrocarbon vapours in the atmosphere have health implications. The effect of formaldehyde is primarily irritating. It is a major contributor to eye and respiratory irritation caused by phtochemical smog.

Carcinogenic Agents

Carcinogenic agents are responsible for cancer. For example, the poly-cyclic organic compounds, 3, 4-benzpyrene. The origin of these compounds is in the incomplete combustion of hydrocarbons and other carbonaceous materials. They are also reported to be present in exhaust discharges from I.C. engines. In addition to poly-cyclic organic compounds, it has been found that some aliphatic hydrocarbons are also carcinogenic.

Insecticides

Insecticides are not only harmful for insects but also poisonous for man, e.g., DDT (Dichloro diphenyl trichloroethane). They can affect the central nervous system and may attack other vital organs. In fact, DDT has been found in mother's milk in western countries and even in our own country. Hence, the use of DDT has been banned in the USA. The United Nations Environment programme (UNEP) has warned against the undesirable effects of indoor spraying of DDT. It has also been reported that indoor spraying effects domestic livestock.

According to a study conducted at the Industrial Toxicology Research Centre, Lucknow (India), the accumulation of pesticides in the environment due to their growing use for agricultural purposes can also cause premature labour and abortion, due to high concentration of pesticides in the body of expectant mothers.

Organic Pollutants, and Photochemical Smog

Hydrocarbons and phtochemical oxidants are two separate, but related, categories of pollutant compounds. Hydrocarbons are primary pollutants, because they get introduced directly into the air. Photochemical oxidants are secondary pollutants producing in the atmosphere form reactions involving primary pollutants. Both groups will be described together because the majority of photochemical oxidants originate from reactions in which hydrocarbons are directly or indirectly involved. Any estimate of the effects of atmosphere hydrocarbon pollution must include the contributions made by phtochemical oxidants. In fact, most of the principal effects of hydrocarbon pollution are brought about by compounds producing from atmospheric reactions of hydrocarbons.

Hydrocarbons Found in the Atmosphere

The number of hydrocarbons involved in air pollution is fairly large. An analysis of urban air by gas chromatography has resulted in the identification of 56 different hydrocarbon compounds. The number present is probably large, but the sensitivity of the analytical method prevented others, in very low concentrations, from being detected.

Natural sources contribute huge quantities of these substance. Plants, particularly trees, emit hydrocarbons. Most of the hydrocarbons emitted to the atmosphere by plants are thought to be *terpanes*. Most of the plants which produce terpenes belong to the family *Coniferae*, the family *Myrtaceace*, and the genus *Citrus*. Isoprene (2-methyl-1, 3-butadiene), a hemiterpene, has been identified in the emissions of cottonwood, eucalyptus, oak, sweetgum, and white spruce trees.

Turpentine, common terpene, is widely used in paint because it reacts with atmospheric oxygen to form a peroxide, then a hard resin. It is likely that compounds such as a-pinene and isoprene undergo similar reactions in the atmosphere to form particulate matter. The resulting Aitken nuclei aerosols probably cause the blue haze associated with the atmosphere above some heavy growths of vegetation.

In addition to the hydrocarbons produced by higher plants, methane is the other major naturally occurring hydrocarbon emitted to the atmosphere. Methane is formed in huge quantities by bacteria in the anaerobic decomposition of organic matter in water, sediments, and soil

$$2CH_2O \xrightarrow{\text{bacteria}} CO_2 + CH_4 \quad ...(1)$$

The fate of atmospheric methane is not known with certainty.

Most of the pollutant hydrocarbons added to the atmosphere through the activities of man are produced by automobiles. Global sources of hydrocarbon emissions are estimated in Table 1. The net air pollution effect of a given source of hydrocarbons is determined by the overall reactivity of hydrocarbons from the source as well as total amount. Most hydrocarbon pollutant sources produce about 15 per cent reactive hydrocarbons, whereas those from gasoline are about 45 per cent reactive.

Table 1

Global and U.S. Emissions of Pollutant Hydrocarbons

Source	*Emissions*
Petroleum	%
Refining	7.2
Oils and distillates	0.4
Gasoline	38.5
Evaporation in transfer and storage	8.8
Coal	
Heating	2.3
Power generation	0.2
Industrial uses	0.8
Wood (fuel and forest fires)	2.2
Incinerators and refuse burning	28.3
Solvent evaporation	11.3

A number of different specific hydrocarbon compounds are found in regions heavily polluted by such substances. Over 20 different compounds were identified and analyzed. Of these, methane was present at by far the highest concentration, an average of 2400 *parts per billion* (ppb) by volume in downtown Los Angeles. Aside from methane, 80% of the remaining hydrocarbons consisted of 10 compounds. These compounds and their average levels were ethane and ethylene (102 ppb total), acetylene and propane (76 ppb total), *n*-butane (46 ppb), isopentane (35 ppb), toluene (30 ppb), *n*-pentane (21 ppb), *m*-xylene (12 ppb), and isobutane (12 ppb). It was observed that as the day progressed the concentration of unsaturated hydrocarbons (butenes) decreased to a greater extent than that of the paraffins. The decrease in the paraffins was attributed entirely to mixing and consequent dilution.

Industrial processes constitute the next largest source. Hydrocarbons get lost to the atmosphere during production, processing storage, and transfer of products containing them. Gasoline hydrocarbons are lost in vapour form during the loading of tank trucks, the filling of service station storage tanks, and the filling of service station storage tanks, and the filling of automobile fuel tanks. The evaporation of organic solvents, most of which contain hydrocarbons, accounts for nearly 10% of all industrial emissions. These solvents are important ingredients of paints, varnishes, lacquers, undercoatings and other similar products. These products consist of 40.80% solvent, which usually evaporates during or after application. The processes involved in the manufacture of these products also comprise potential hydrocarbon sources.

The gasoline powered automobile is the major culprit in producing pollutant hydrocarbons. At the high temperatures and pressures encountered in the automobile engine, gasoline which is not completely burned undergoes chemical reactions which produce several hundred kinds of hydrocarbons. Some of these are highly reactive in the atmosphere, and others, such as benzopyrene, are known carcinogens. These hydrocarbons spew from automobile exhausts into the faces of pedestrians and drift upward in the atmosphere where, with the help of solar energy, they are cooked into an even more exotic mixture of photochemical oxidation products above our cities. It is little wonder, therefore, that the control of automotive hydrocarbons has had the top priority in the effort to acquire clean air.

Aside from the exhust, the automobile contains several potential sources of pollutant hydrocarbons (Fig. 1). One source is the crankcase, which is having mist composed of lubricating oil, and receives "blowby" consisting of exhaust gas and unoxidized carbureted mixture from around the pistons. Blowby is recirculated through the engine intake manifold by way of the PCV (positive crankcase ventilation) valve. These emissions were the first to be controlled.

The fuel system has been a second major source of automotive hydrocarbon emissions. Fuel may be given off through fuel tank and carburetor vents. When the engine is shut down and engine heat worms up the fuel system, gasoline may be evaporated and emitted to the atmosphere. In addition, hearing during the daytime and cooling at night causes the fuel tank to breathe and emit gasoline fumes.

Many systems have been devised for the control of evaporative emissions from fuel systems. One is a carbon canister which is able to collect evaporated fuel from the fuel tank and fuel system, to be purged and burned when the engine is operating. Reduction of fuel volatility also helps cut down hydrocarbon evaporation from fuel systems. The automobile exhaust is the greatest source of hydrocarbons. They are produced by the engine, which for the vast majority of automobiles is a fourcycle internal combustion engine fueled with gasoline. The four basic steps in the complete cycle of the engine are the following:

1. *Intake.* An air-gasoline mixture formed in the carbouretor and consisting of about 14-15 parts by weight of air per part gasoline gets drawn into the cylinder through the open intake valve.

2. *Compression.* The combustible mixture gets compressed by a ratio of about 8.5 :1. Higher compression ratios tend to favour thermal efficiency and complete combustion of hydrocarbons. However, higher temperature, premature combustion ("pingin"), and high production of nitrogen oxides also result from higher combustion ratios.

3. *Ignition and power stroke.* As the fuel-air mixture gets ignited by a spark plug near top-dead-center of the combustion stroke, a temperature of about 2500°C is reached very rapidly at pressures up to 40 atm. The temperature decreases in a few milliseconds. This rapid cooling "freezes" nitric oxide in the form of NO without permitting it time to dissociate to N_2 and O_2, thermodynamically favoured at the temperature and pressure of the atmosphere.

4. *Exhaust.* Exhaust gases having largely of N_2 and CO_2 with trace of CO, NO, hydrocarbons, and O_2 get pushed out through the open exhaust valve, thus completing the cycle.

The primary cause of hydrocarbons in the exhaust gas has been "wall quench." The relatively cool wall in the combustion chamber of the internal combustion engine quenches the flame within several thousandths of an inch of the wall. Part of the remaining hydrocarban may get retained as residual gas in the cylinder, and part may get oxidized in the exhaust system. The remainder goes to the atmosphere as pollutant hydrocarbons. Engine misfire due to the improper adjustment and decleration greatly tends to increase the emissions of hydrocarbons. Turbine engines are not subject to the wall quench phenomenon because their surfaces are always hot.

Several engine design characteristics favour low exhaust hydrocarbon emissions. Spark retard reduces exhaust hydrocarbon emissions. One reason for this reduction is that the effective surface/volume ratio of the combustion chamber is reduced. Secondly, when the spark is retarded, the combustion products are purged from the cylinders sooner after combustion. Therefore, the exhaust gas is hotter, and reactions consuming hydrocarbons get promoted in the exhaust system.

The "air pump" or "Thermactor" is used to control hydrocarbon as well as carbon monoxide emissions. A more sophisticated device similar to the Thermactor is the thermal exhaust reactor which is insulated and provides a large volume in which exhaust gases can be retained for some time to react at high temperature with fresh air pumped into the system. Many catalytic exhaust reactors have been devised for the oxidation of excess hydrocarbons. For the control of hydrocarbons and carbon monoxide, these catalytic reactors require an excess of oxygen, whereas for the removal of NO_x a reducing atmosphere is required. Therefore, two beds of catalyst are required.

Catalytic exhaust reactors using platinum catalysts came into widespread use in the United States during the 1975 model year. Since lead poisons the catalyst used, the automobiles equipped with catalytic exhaust control devices require lead-free gasoline, and facilities for dispensing this fuel have been installed in all major service stations. Recent evidence also suggests that catalytic exhaust reactors result in the production of potentially hazardous levels of sulfuric acid by catalysis of the oxidation of sulfur dioxide from sulfur-containing gasoline:

$$2SO_2 + O_2 \rightarrow 2SO_3 \qquad ...(1)$$

$$SO_3 + H_2O \rightarrow H_2SO_4 \qquad ...(2)$$

Photochemical Oxidants

The term *photochemical oxidant* is used to describe an atmospheric substance, produced by a photochemical process (a chemical process that requires light), which will oxidize materials not readily oxidized by gaseous oxygen. These substances are secondary pollutants produced by an interaction of primary pollutants with light.

Hydrocarbons are very much involved in the production of photochemical oxidants. The large variety of hydrocarbons involved in these reactions prevents a simple explanation from being formulated for the various processes. Although the intimate details of the reactions are not known, several specific facts are known quite well. The involvement of the NO_2 photolytic cycle has been definitely established. Two of the most harmful secondary pollutants produced as a result of the involvement of hydrocarbons in this cycle have been identified. These are ozone (O_3), a form of oxygen and peroxyacetylnitrate, the simplest member of a group of a compounds, peroxyactylnitrates, usually referred to collectively as PAN.

Ozone is obviously not a hydrocarbon, but its concentration increase in the atmosphere is a direct result of hydrocarbon reaction PAN is seen to be a hydrocarbon derivative.

Formation of Photochemical Oxidants

The majority of the harmful effects of hydrocarbon pollution are not caused by the hydrocarbons themselves, but by the products of photochemical reactions in which the dydrocarbons are involved. Hydrocarbons do not readily react with sunlight, but they are reactive toward other substances produced photochemically. The photolytic cycle of NO generate several material with which hydrocarbons readily react. The NO_2 cycle involves the three reactions:

$$NO_2 + \text{Sunlight} \rightarrow NO + O \qquad ...(1)$$

$$O + O_2 \rightarrow O_3 \qquad ...(2)$$

$$O_3 + NO \rightarrow NO_2 + O_2 \qquad ...(3)$$

and the net effect should be a rapid cycling of NO_2. Ozone (O_3) and NO should be formed and destroyed equal quantities.

The cycle gets distrupted when hydrocarbons are present because of their ability to react with either the oxygen atoms (O) produced (equation 1) or the ozone produced (equation 2). The most likely reaction is that between O and hydrocarbons, because it takes place 10^8 times faster than the one between O_3 and hydrocarbons. The reaction between O and O_2 is faster than that between oxygen atoms and hydrocarbons, but the latter reaction still proceeds fast enough to upset the cycle.

The product of a reaction between O and a hydrocarbon is a very reactive intermediate species called a hydrocarbon free radical (RO_2). Free radicals of this type can further react with a number of different species including NO, NO_2, O, O_2, O_3, and other hydrocarbons. Some general facts are known.

1. The free radicals react rapidly with NO to produce NO_2. The consequence of this is that with NO removed from the cycle, the normal mechanism for O_3 removal (equation 3) has been eliminated, and the concentration of O_3 in air gets increased.
2. The free radicals can react with O_2 and N_2 to give peroxyacylnitrate (PAN).
3. The free radicals can react with other hydrocarbons and oxygen species to produce additional undesirable organic compounds.

These interactions, resulting from the disruption of the NO_2 photolytic cycle by hydrocarbons. The mixture of products resulting from the hydrocarbon interference in the NO_2 photolytic cycle is called photochemical smog. It consists of occumulated O_3, CO, PAN, and other organic compounds, including aldehydes, ketones, and alkyl nitrates.

There is a wide variation in the tendency for different hydrocarbons to enter into the photochemical air pollution process. As a consequence, it is impossible to predict accurately, on the basis of total hydrocarbon concentration, the contribution of a hydrocarbon mixture to photochemical air pollution. The detailed composition of the mixture must be known.

Importance of Hydrocarbon Pollution

Except in cases of very severe contamination, generally involving polycyclic aromatic hydrocarbons, atmospheric hydrocarbons in themselves are not severe air pollutants. However, hydrocarbons entering the atmosphere as primary pollutants produce photochemical oxidants as secondary pollutants. These oxidants give rise to a number of undesirable effects such as the notorious smog which afflicts Los Angeles and other urban areas. Atmospheric oxidants cause eye and respiratory tract irritation and are suspected of imparing human health. Some plants have been very susceptible to damage by oxidants. One such oxidant is ozone, O_3. Chemically, ozone is of course entirely different from the hydrocarbons which are required for its formation in low level atmospheres. Other oxidants like peroxyacetyl-nitrate, PAN, differ a great deal chemically from their hydrocarbon precursors.

Reactions of Hydrocarbons in the Atmosphere

Hydrocarbons undergo chemical and photochemical reactions in the atmosphere. With carbon monoxide as a nonreactive standard for pollutant emissions, the expected levels of hydrocarbons in the atmosphere may be calculated from the known composition of pollutant sources.

The photochemical reactions are able to initiate most of the chemical processes culminating in removal of hydrocarbons from the atmosphere. The most important of these primary photochemical reactions in an atmosphere is

$$NO_2 + h\nu \rightarrow NO + O \qquad ...(1)$$

whereby nitrogen dioxide undergoes photochemical dissociation to yield NO and atomic oxygen. The second most important primary photochemical reaction probably involves the formation of free radicals from aldehydes:

$$CH_3 - \overset{\overset{\displaystyle O}{\|}}{C}\text{-}H + h\nu \rightarrow CH_2 + H - CO \qquad ...(2)$$

It is possible that in some atmospheres other primary photochemical processes may be more important than the above.

In addition to aldehydes, compounds forming free radicals in the atmosphere include ketones, organic peroxides, organic nitrates, and hydrogen peroxide. Free radicals certainly are also involved in the reactions of atmospheric hydrocarbons. For example, it has been hypothesized that the initial reaction of *n*-butane by photolysis in an atmosphere containing NO_2 is the reaction the paraffin with atomic oxygen [produced by Reaction (1)].

$$C_4H_{10} + O \rightarrow C_4H_9 + OH \quad ...(3)$$

Free radicals may react with other species to form other radicals. For example, the *n*-butyl radical formed in Reaction (3) is thought to react with molecular oxygen to from a peroxy radical:

$$C_4H_9 + O_2 \rightarrow C_4H_9OO. \quad ...(4)$$

Hydroxyl radicals may be formed from the peroxy radical by the following reaction:

$$C_4H_9OO \rightarrow \underset{\text{methyl ethyl keton}}{CH_3CH_2CCH_3} + OH \quad ...(5)$$

The hydroxyl radical may react with additional *n*-butane

$$C_4H_{10} + OH \rightarrow C_4H_9 + H_2O \quad ...(6)$$

to form more *n*-butyl radical. The *n*-butyl radical may participate in Reaction (4). Thus Reactions (4) through (6) constitute a chain in which hydroxyl radical is the chain-propagating free radical.

The above reactions demonstrate some of the more important aspects of free radical reactions which are involving hydrocarbon in the atmosphere. There is first of all a *primary photochemical reaction,* in this case the phtotodissociation of NO_2 to NO and atomic oxygen,

Reaction (1). Next comes a *chain-initiating reaction,* in this case the reaction of atomic oxygen with *n*-butane, Reaction (3). The chain of Reactions (4) through (6) may continue until the chain-propagating free radical is destroyed in a *chain-terminating step.* Chain termination may take place in several ways, including reaction of two free radicals,

$$2OH \rightarrow H_2 + O \qquad ...(7)$$

adduct formation with nitric oxide or nitrogen dioxide,

$$OH + NO_2 + M \rightarrow HNO_3 + M \qquad ...(8)$$

(Here M refers to a third body which absorbs energy), or reaction of the radical with a solid particle surface.

Gas phase reaction chains may have as many as one million steps. Furthermore, chain-branching reactions in which a free radical reacts with an excited molecule making it to produce two new free radicals may occur.

Free radicals are quite reactive: therefore, they generally have short lifetimes. Hydrocarbons may undergo heterogeneous reactions on particles in the atmosphere.

Dusts composed of metal oxides or charcoal are having a catalytic effect upon the oxidation of organic compounds. Metal oxides may enter into photochemical reactions.

For example, zinc oxide photosensitized by exposure to light has been found to promote oxidation of organic compounds

Oxidants in the Atomsphere: Phtochemical Smog

An oxidant in air pollution parlance of a substance in the atmosphere capable of oxidizing iodide ion to iodine (O).

Sometimes substances other than iodide ion are used as reducing agents in the measurement of oxidants.

A number of diffferent compounds—including O_3, NO_2, H_2O_2, organic peroxides, orgnic hydroperoxides, and peroxycyl nitrate—are oxidants in the atmosphere. Organic peroxides are having the general formula ROOR', and organic hydroperoxides are having the formula ROOH.

Probably, the most notorious organic oxidant has been peroxyacetyl nitrate, PAN which has the formula as follows:

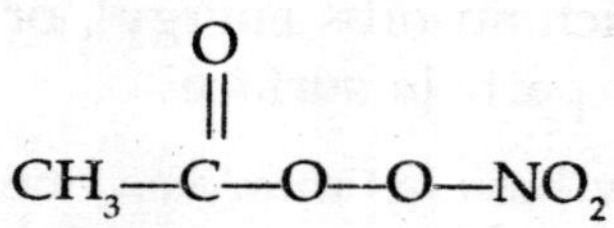

PAN, as well as other member of its homologous series of compounds, is produced photochemically in atmospheres having olefins and NO_x. It is damaging to plants, attacking younger leaves and bringng about "bronzing" and "glazing" of their surfaces.

Exposure for several hours to an atmosphere containing PAN at a level of only 0.02 to 0.05 ppm will damge vegetation.

The sulfhydryl group on proteins has been susceptible to damage by PAN. In reacting with sulfhydryl groups PAN may act as both an oxidizing agent and an acetylating agent.

Peroxybenzoyl nitrate, PBN, occurs in polluted atmospheres. It is a powerful eye irritant and lachrymator. It may be produced in the atmosphere by photochemical reactions which are involving aromatic hydrocarbons, nitrogen oxides and ozone.

In addition to PAN and PBN, some other specific organic oxidants which may be important in polluted atmospheres include peroxypropinyl nitrate (PPN) ; peracetic acid, $CH_3(CO)OOH$; acetylperoxide, $CH_3(CO)OO(CO)CH_3$; ethyl hydroperoxide, CH_3CH_2OOH; n-butylhydroperoxide, $CH_3CH_2CH_2COOH$; and *tert*-butylhydroperoxide, $(CH_3)_3$ COOH.

During the 1940s the Los Angeles area in California began experiencing a new and serious form of air pollution which was characterized by reduced visibility and eye irritation. The term "smog" has since been used to describe this kind of air pollution. The term is a misnomer for it was originally used to describe the unpleasant combination of smoke and fog laced with sulfur dioxide formerly very prevalent in London. However, either smoke or fog nhibits the formation of photochemical smog of the Los Angeles type. These two types of smog are in many ways exact opposites in their chemical behaviour. The mixture of smoke, fog, and sulfur dioxide which afflicted London so badly for several centuries after the introduction of coal as a fuel is chemically a reducing mixture and is termed as a *reducing smog*. The smog which permeates the Los Angeles area of number of days each year has a high concentration of oxidants and is an oxidizing mixture. It is therefore termed as an *oxidizing smog*. Of course, readily oxidized sulfur dioxide cannot last long in an atmosphere where oxidizing photochemical smog is present.

In this section are discussed some of the primary aspects of photochemical smog formation.

The formation of oxidants in the air—particularly ozone, but including PAN and other—has been indicative of smog formation. Serious levels of photochemical smog may be assumed to be present when the oxidant level exceeds 0.15 ppm for more than one hour. Ultraviolet light initiates smog formation and photochemical processes are involved. Hydrocarbons must be present, and olefins are especially conductive to smog formation. Nitrogen oxides are required for the formation of smog, and a level of approximate 0.15 ppm NO_x is optimum. Apparently nitrogen oxides are involved in the primary photochemical processes leading to smog formation. As it has been established that nitrogen oxides can inhibit atmospheric photooxidation of hydrocarbons, probably by queening reactions involving free radaicals (see Reaction 8), some concern exists that partial success in reducing nitrogen oxide emissions in some localities might actually increase the incidence of smog.

Smoggy atmospheres show characteristic variations with time of day in levels of NO, NO_2, hydrocarbons, aldehydes, and oxidants.

The time-variations in levels of hydrocarbons, ozone, NO, and NO_2 are explained in a group of overall reactions first proposed by Friedlander and Seinfeld:

1. Primary photochemical reaction:

$$NO_2 + hv \rightarrow NO + O \qquad ...(1)$$

2. Reactions involving oxygen species :

$$O_2 + O + M \rightarrow O_3 + M \qquad ...(2)$$

(M is an energy-absorbing third body)

$$O_3 + NO \rightarrow NO_2 + O_2 \qquad ...(3)$$

3. Production of organic free radicals from hydrocarbons, RH :

$$O + RH \rightarrow R. + \text{other products} \qquad ...(4)$$

$$O_3 + RH \rightarrow R. \text{ and/or other products} \qquad ...(5)$$

R. is a free radical which may, or may not, contain oxygen.

4. *Chain propagation, branching and termination:*

$$NO + R. \rightarrow NO_2 + R \qquad ...(6)$$

In this case R contains oxygen and oxidizes NO. It is one of many chain propagation [reaction, some of which involve NO.]

$$NO_2 + R. \rightarrow \text{products (e.g., PAN)}$$

This is the most common chain terminating reaction, which occurs because NO_2 is a stable free radical present at high concentrations in a smoggy atmosphere. Reaction with NO may also occur. Chains may be terminated by reaction of two R. radicals, although this is uncommon because of their relatively low concentrations. Radical sorption on a particle surface is also possible and may contribute to particle growth.

Many specific reactions are involved in the above overall scheme for the formation of photochemical smog. The formation of atomic oxygen by the primary photochemical reaction

$$NO_2 + hv \rightarrow NO + O \qquad ...(7)$$

leads to several reactions involving oxygen and nitrogen oxide species:

$$O + O_2 + M \rightarrow O_3 + M \qquad ...(8)$$

$$O + NO + M \rightarrow NO_2 + M\cdot \qquad ..(9)$$

$$O + NO_2 \rightarrow NO + O_2 \qquad ...(10)$$

$$O_3 + NO \rightarrow NO_2 + O_2 \qquad ...(11)$$

$$O + NO_2 + M \rightarrow NO_3 + M \qquad ...(12)$$

$$O_3 + NO_2 \rightarrow NO_3 + O_2 \qquad ...(13)$$

There are a number of significant atmospheric reactions involving nitrogen oxides, water, nitrous acid, and nitiric acid:

$$NO_3 + NO_2 \rightarrow N_2O_5 \qquad ...(14)$$

$$NO_3 + NO \rightarrow 2NO_2 \qquad ...(15)$$

$$NO_3 + NO_2 \rightarrow N_2O_5 \qquad ...(16)$$

[The reverse of Reaction (16) also occurs in a significant extent.]

$$N_2O_5 + HO \rightarrow 2HNO_3 \qquad ...(17)$$

(Some of the nitiric acid produced in Reaction 17 may react with ammonia or particulate basic material to form particulate nitrates, which cause severe corrosion problems to, for example, electrical relay contacts.)

$$NO + HNO_3 \rightarrow HNO_2 + NO_2 \qquad ...(18)$$

$$HNO_2 + HNO_3 \rightarrow H_2O + 2NO_2 \qquad ...(19)$$

$$NO + NO_2 + H_2O \rightarrow 2HNO_2 \qquad ...(20)$$

$$2HNO_2 \rightarrow NO + NO_2 + H_2O \qquad ...(21)$$

Very reactive hydroxyl radicals, HO, can be formed by the reaction of excited atomic oxygen with water,

$$O + H_2O \rightarrow 2HO \qquad ...(22)$$

photodissociation of hydrogen peroxide,

$$H_2O_2 + hv \rightarrow 2HO \qquad ...(23)$$

or by the photolysis of nitrous acid,

$$HNO_2 + hv \rightarrow HO + NO \qquad ...(24)$$

Among the inorganic species with which the hydroxyl radical reacts are oxides of nitrogen.

$$HO + NO_2 \rightarrow HNO_3 \qquad ...(25)$$

$$HO + NO + M \rightarrow HNO_2 + M \qquad ...(26)$$

and carbon monoxide,

$$CO + HO + O_2 \rightarrow CO_2 + HO_2 \qquad ...(27)$$

The last reaction is significant in that it may be responsible for the disappearance of some atmospehric CO and because it produces the hydroperoxy radical HO_2. One of the major inorganic reactions of the hydroperoxy radical is the oxidation of NO :

$$HO_2 + NO \rightarrow HO + NO_2 \qquad ...(28)$$

The kinetic rate constants for most of the above reactions are reasonably well known, enabling calculations of species concentrations to be expected under various conditions. These calculations, supported by laboratory studies of irradiated mixtures, are not able to explain the rapid transformation of NO and NO_2 that occurs in an atmosphere undergoing photochemical smog formation. In fact, except at very high CO concentration the concentration of NO_2 is predicted to remain at very low levels. However, in the presence of reactive hydrocarbons, NO_2 accumulates very rapidly by a reaction process beginning with its photodissociation. It can be concluded, therefore, that the organic compounds form species which react with NO directly, rather than with NO_2.

Aliphatic hydrocarbons, RH, can react with O,

$$RH + O + O_2 \rightarrow ROO. + HO \qquad ...(29)$$

or HO radical,

$$RH + HO + O_2 \rightarrow ROO. + H_2O \qquad ..(30)$$

to produce relative oxygenated organic radicals, ROO. Olefins R = R' are much more reactive, undergoing overall reactions such as the following:

$$R = R' + O + 2O_2 \rightarrow ROO. + R''\overset{\overset{O}{\|}}{C}OO. \qquad ...(31)$$

$$R = R' + O + 2O_2 \rightarrow ROO. + HO_2 + CO \qquad ...(32)$$

(In reactions such as 32 and 38 below where the HCO radical is formed, the HCO radical is believed to react with O_2 to form CO and H_2O radical.)

$$R = R' + HO = O \rightarrow ROO. + H\overset{\overset{O}{\|}}{C}R'' \text{ (an aldehyde)} \qquad ..(33)$$

Aromatic hydrocarbons, H, may also react with O and HO :

$$\varnothing H + O + O_2 \rightarrow \varnothing OO. + H_2O \qquad ...(34)$$

$$\varnothing H + HO + O_2 \rightarrow \varnothing OO. + H_2O \qquad ...(35)$$

Aldehydes, $H\overset{\overset{O}{\|}}{C}R''$, react with HO,

$$H\overset{\overset{O}{\|}}{C}R'' + HO + O_2 \rightarrow R''\overset{\overset{O}{\|}}{C}OO. + H_2O \qquad ...(36)$$

$$H_2C = O + HO + 3/2O_2 \rightarrow CO_2 + H_2\dot{O} + H_2O \qquad ...(37)$$

(formaldehyde)

and undergo photochemical reactions:

$$H\overset{\overset{O}{\|}}{C}R'' + hv + 2O_2 \rightarrow R''OO. + CO + HO_2 \qquad ...(38)$$

$$H_2C = O + hv\ 2O_2 \rightarrow CO = 2HO_2 \qquad ...(39)$$

From the above reactions it is seen that hydrocarbons reacting with atomic oxygen or hydroxyl groups produce oxygen-containing free radical which are highly reactive. The reactions of these radicals with NO

$$ROO. + NO \rightarrow RO. + NO_2 \qquad ...(40)$$

$$R\overset{\overset{\displaystyle O}{\|}}{C}OO. + NO + O_2 \rightarrow ROO. + NO_2 + CO_2 \qquad ...(41)$$

are responsible for the rapid conversion of NO to NO_2. Peroxyacyl nitrates (PAN) are formed by an addition reaction with $NO_{2:}$

$$R\overset{\overset{\displaystyle O}{\|}}{C}OO. + NO_2 \downarrow R\overset{\overset{\displaystyle O}{\|}}{C}OONO_2 \qquad ...(42)$$

Alkyl nitrates and alkyl nitrites may be formed by the reaction of alkoxyl radicals (RO.) with nitrogen dioxide and nitric oxide respectively:

$$RO. + NO_2 \rightarrow RONO_2 \qquad ...(43)$$

$$RO. + NO \rightarrow RONO \qquad ...(44)$$

Addition reactions with NO_2 such as these are important in terminating the reaction chain involved in smog formation. Since NO_2 is involved both in the chain initiation step (Reaction 1) and the chain termination step, it is unlikely that moderate reductions in NO_x emissions alone will have much influence on curtailing smog formation. The reaction of oxygen with alkoxyl radicals

$$RO. + O_2 \rightarrow HO_2 + H\overset{\overset{\displaystyle O}{\|}}{C}R'' \qquad ...(45)$$

produces hydroperoxy radical. Peroxy radicals are able to react with one another.

$$HO_2 + HO_2 \rightarrow H_2O_2 + O_2 \quad ...(46)$$

$$HO_2 + ROO. \rightarrow RO. + HO + O_2 \quad ..(47)$$

$$ROO. + ROO. \rightarrow 2RO_2 + O_2 \quad ...(48)$$

to produce reactive hydrogen peroxide, alkoxyl radicals and hydroxyl radicals.

Recently it is argued that electronically excited singlet oxygen designated here as O_2* (g), may be an important oxidizing agent in the atmosphere, and contribute to the atmospheric oxidation of NO to NO_2. The abosrption of light by ground-state oxygen, O_2 (3Σg) takes place in the wavelength regiouns of 687 nm and 759 to 766 nm. The absorption is too weak to account for any appreciable level of singlet oxygen in the atmosphere. However, oxygen may be excited to the singlet state by energy transfer from another excited species.

Ultraviolet irradiation of mixtures of benzaldehyde and oxygen has produced singlet oxygen as evidenced by its emission of light of 1.27 micron wavelength. Although it has not been established that singlet oxygen participates significantly in atmospheric oxidation processes, it is known to react with olefins for forming peroxidic organic compounds. These compounds could then decompose to form radicals of the type RCO, thus starting the chain reaction process involved in smog formation.

Aerosol particles are formed by the polymerization of the smaller molecules which are produced in the primary smog forming reactions. The chemical composition of the aerosol particles shows a high percentage of oxygen. Ether-soluble aerosols collected from the Los Angeles atmosphere show an empirical formula of approximately CH_2O. Therefore, the original hydrocarbons are strongly oxidized by reactions in the atmosphere.

London Smog

That there is a fundamental connection between air pollution and damge to health has been recognized for many years. Doctors, scientists and public health centers were altered to the problem when serious smog disasters occurred in the valley of the River Maas in Belgium in 1930 and in the city centre of Donora in the United States in 1948. Many people died as a result, and the coincidence in time of the atmospheric pollution and the resulting health damage highlighted the causes of the maladies and deaths.

Considerably more action for the reduction of atmospheric pollution was promoted by the occurrence of fog in London. From December 5 to 9, 1952, many regions in Great britain were cloaked in fog. Particularly affected was the wide valley of the river Thames with London in its midst. Within about 12 hours of the appearance of the heavy fog (which owing to a sharp inversion of weather conditions entrapped all the waste gases from the city), an extremely large number of people in London were smitten with breathing difficulties. This was soon followed by an unusually high number of deaths.

The symptoms of the malady were severe coughing and expectoration, increased nasal secretions, sore throats and sudden vomitting. Generally speaking the troubles began without warming. Many of the most serious cases, mainly people already suffering from chronic bronchitis, asthma or pulmonary fibrosis, occurred on the third or fourth day of fog. The symptoms of patients seriously affected were shortness of breadth, cyanosis, fever, rattling in the throat and bronchospasms. A subsequent assessment of the mortality figures revealed that in 14 days of the smog disaster 4000 more people died altogether than was normal in the period.

From the very first day of the catastrophe, the number of deaths increased significantly; and the increase was greater in the center of London than in the outer ring of the city. A further 4000 people died in the following weeks and months. All age groups were affected, but those over 45 years of age and babies of up to 1 year most severely. In the age group from 1 to 14 years the death rate during the smog catastrophe was 1.3 times the previous rate, for over 45 year olds 2.8 times, and for babies 2.2 times.

During the smog disaster the concentration of sulfur dioxide in the atmosphere amounted on the average to 0.7 ppm, or about 6 times the normal level. The smoke concentration was about 5 times the normal. At that time it was still assumed that such a level was medically harmless. Subsequently, a number of other cases of smog occurred in London: January 3 to 6, 1956 (1000 deaths); December 2 to 5, 1957 (800); December 5 to 10, 1962 (700); and January 7 to 22, 1963 (700). It was only after these further catastrophes, in which thousands more victims perished, that atmospheric pollution over London was severely cut back by intensive counter-measures so that the danger of serious smog disasters in London now seems to have been averted. By a change in heating techiques and by insisting on the use of smokeless fuels, the hours of sunshine in winter have been raised in London by 70%.

Injury to vegetation was one of the earliest observed results of photochemical air pollution. Available information suggests that ozone is the most toxic photochemical to plants, but continuing research is uncovering the importance of the PAN family. The effects of ozone on some particular plants are given in Table 2.

Table 2

Toxic Effects of Ozone on Plants

Plant	*Ozone Level (ppm)*	*Exposure Time*	*Observed Effects*
Radish	0.05	20 days (8-hr/day)	50% reduction in yield
Carnation	00.7	60 days	50% reduction in floral development
Tobacco	0.10	5-5 hours	50% reduction in pollen germination and pollen tube growth

Visible effects of ozone injure to plants are bleached or light flecks of stipples (small clusters of dead cells on the upper surface of leaves. Fully expanded, mature leaves are most easily damaged. Emergence tip burn, a disease of white pine, puzzled foresters and plant pathologists for years. It has been found that the presence of ozone correlates with the occurrence of this disease.

The other major secondary photochemical pollutant is peroxyacetylnitrate. Other common peroryacylnitrates are peroxypropionylnitrate (PPN), peroxybutyrylnitrate (PBN) and peroxyisobutyrylnitrate ($P_{iso}BN$). Preliminary studies show than PPN is several times as toxic to plants as PAN, while PBN and $P_{iso}BN$ are still more toxic than PPN.

Plant injury from PAN shows up as a glazing and bronzing of the lower leaf surfaces and a general attack on younger leaves. Eventually, leaf tissue dies. Exposures of a few hours to PAN concentrations of 0.02 to 0.05 ppm are sufficient to cause injury to vegetation. Five hours of exposure to a PAN level of 0.01 ppm will injure the most sensitive plants. It has been found especially toxic to citrus, forage and salad crops, and coniferous trees. Ethylene (CH) is the only hydrocarbon known to have adverse effects on vegetation at ambient concentrations of 1 ppm or, less. Acetylence and propylene have shown some toxicity toward plants but only at concentrations of from 60-500 times as high as that of ethylene. The principal effect of ethylene upon plants is inhibition of growth. It also brings about color changes in leaves and death of flowering parts.

Currently, there is no evidence to indicate that hydrocarbons, at present ambient air concentrations, exert any direct undesirable effects on humans. Experimental data obtained from research on humans and animals indicate that acyclic and alicyclic hydrocarbons produce undesirable effects only at concentrations hundreds to thousands of times higher than those now found in the atmosphere. No effects have been reported for levels lower than 500 ppm. Aromatic hydrocarbons are a greater threat than the acyclinc alicyclic. The vapours are much more irritating to the mucous membranes, and systemic injury can result from the inhalation of aromatic compound vapours. However, no effects have been reported at air concentrations lower than 25 ppm. Some effects of two common aromatics are given in Table 3.

Photochemical oxidants enter the body as part of inhaled air and at sublethal concentrations alter, impair of otherwise interfere with normal respiratory processes. Some eye irritation is also characteristic of exposure to these compounds.

The following effects have been observed in humans exposed to ozone under experimental conditions: in general, no ill effects were noted at concentrations up to

0.2 ppm and a level of about 0.3 ppm appeared to be the threshold level at which nose and throat irritation began. Specifically, exposure to ozone concentrations of 1.0 to 3.0 ppm for a period of 2 hours produced extreme fatigue and lack of coordination in sensitive experimental subjects. Exposure to concentrations of about 9.0 ppm for similar time periods produced severe pulmonary edema in most subjects.

Table 3

Toxicity of two Aromatic Hydrocarbons

Compound	*Concentration (ppm)*	*Effect*
Benzene	100	Mucous membrane irritation.
C_6H_6	3,000	Endurable 1/2 hour.
	7,500	Dangerous after 1/2 hour
	20,000	Fetal after 5-10 minutes.
Toluene	200	Mild fatigue, weakness, and
C_7H_8		confusion after 8 hours.
	600	Loss of coordination, pupils
		dilated after 8 hours.

It appears that at the concentrations known to occur in ambient atmospheres, PAn (peroxyacetylnitrate) does not present any recognized health hazard. It has been linked to eye irritation, but it appears to play only a minor role. Another member of the family, peroxybenzoylnitrate, more readily brings about eye irritation.

Some researchers feel that much of the degradation of materials now attributed to "weathering" is actually the result of attack by air pollutants, particularly photochemical oxidants. Most of the research in this area has dealt with one oxidant, ozone, and two types of materials, rubber and textiles. It is known that many organic polymers, including rubber and natural and synthetic textiles, are subject to chemical alteration upon exposure to very small amounts of ozone. Ambient air concentrations are frequently high enough to cause these reactions to take place. The susceptibility to attack increases with increasing numbers of carbon-to-carbon double bonds in the material. The double bond is the site of such attacks.

Two different effects are produced by these reactions, carbon-chain breaking and carbon-chain cross-linking. In the first, the long chains of carbon atoms that make up the polymer are broken, and the material becomes more fluid-like and loses tensile strength. The second effect results in the formation of new links between parallel carbon chains. This causes the material to become less elastic and more brittle. This type of activity takes place in ambient ozone levels much lower than those known to affect humans.

Rubber in a relaxed state can be exposed to ozone for long periods of time without forming any characteristic cracks. However, exposure to ambient concentrations of 0.01–0.02 ppm ozone will result in the formation of cracks if the rubber is under a strain of as little as 2 or 3%. Apparently, rubber is protected by a coating consisting of a compound of rubber and ozone (ozonide) which forms on the surface and protects against further penetration and attack by ozone. This protective film cracks when the rubber is stretched and fresh rubber surfaces are exposed to the atmospheric ozone.

The main use of rubber is in automobile tires and such rubber is exposed to atmospheric ozone while in a state of continual tensile stress (stretching and flexing). In order to prevent ozone attack and subsequent cracking antiozonant additives are additives are added to the rubber. These prevent ozone attack but quite expensive, costing about 0.50 per tire. Table 4 shows the effects of ozone on unprotected rubber. The rubber strips were in a state of contant strain by being permanently bent during the experiments.

Table 4

Effects of Ozone on Rubber

Concentration of Ozone (ppm)	*Time for First Crack to Appear (Minutes)*
0.02	65
0.26	5
0.45	3
20,000 (2%)	1 second, cracks formed instantly

Ozone also attacks the cellulose in textile fabrics. Light and humidity appear to be factors necessary before any appreciable alteration takes place in the fiber-breaking strength, The harmful effects of ozone exposure on textiles increases in order for fabrics made of cotton, acetate, nylon, and polyester.

Effects of Oil from Various Sources

Clearly the opportunities to study the effects of oil presented by continuous natural seepage, refinery effluent, oil rig discharges, etc., on the one hand, and the more massive short-term injections of oil arising from oil rig blowouts and tanker accidents on the other, are different, and differences exist even within these two broad classes. It may therefore by though that results obtained in one case may not be applicable in the others. It is thus worthwhile to consider types differences and to assess the extent to which results obtained at the various sites and incidents may be of universal application.

The first point to note in this endeavour is that oil does not dissolve in water. It floats on the sea surface as a thin layer when spilled or otherwise discharged because it is less dense than water and insoluble in it. This thin layer tends to break into droplets by wave action and these droplets become dispersed in the volume of sea water beneath the slick. Photochemical and biological oxidation of the sicks and of the dispersed oil droplets take place producing oxygenated derivatives of the original oil components and these may form true solutions in water.

Thus the area of sea covered by the surface slick is proportional to the magnitude of the spillage, but the concentrations in the sea arise from the slow dispersion of droplets of oxygenated derivatives. Sea water concentrations are therefore a function of mass transfer rates from slick to water and not a function of the quantity spilled. Sea water concentrations are in fact independent of the quantity spilled, provided a surface layer has formed above the sea water volume in question. If more or less oil is spilled or otherwise introduced to the sea the result is more or less sea affected rather than that a given volume is affected to a greater or lesser extent.

Oil concentrations are therefore controlled by the in solubility of the oil and mass transfer rates from surface slicks to the underlying sea. In the absence of detailed knowledge of mass transfer rates it is not possible to calculate the resulting concentrations, but upper limits can easily be established. Thus if the slick thickness to which the oil spreads and from which it subsequently disperses to the water is 0.1 mm, then the maximum concentration which can achieved if the oil were instantaneously dispersed uniformly in the top metre of sea would be 100 ppm. Concentrations over other depth ranges and for other thicknesses are of course pro data.

It must be concluded therefore that is we leave aside for the time being the possible environmental effects of continuous oil slicks on the sea surface which occur when the capacity of the aqueous phase for oil is exceeded, we can discuss the other oil concentration-related aspects in the same manner whether a surface slick is present or not and whether the oil in question acrose from a natural seep, a blowout, cargo tank rupture or operational discharge from ship, oil rig or refinery. Generally speaking, we have limited our discussions to those materials introduced into the marine environment that are the direct result of man's activities, and with a few minor exceptions we shall continue to limit our discussions of pollution to those activities of man and to consider the deleterious effects of natural occurrences.

Pollutant Types

There are three basic type of pollutants: the pathogenic, the aesthetic, and the ecomorphic. Pathogenic pollutants are those which cause disease. This disease may be fatal if the pollutant is a lethal poison.

Aesthetic pollutants are those pollutants causing a change in the environment displeasing to the eye, ear, or nose of man. Ecomorphic pollutants, on the other hand, are those pollutants which produce a change in the physical characteristics of the environment in such a way that there may be drastic changes in the structure or composition of the biosphere.

Obviously, these three types of pollutants are not of equal import. Pathogenic pollutants are certainly much more serious than the other two; however, ecomorphic pollutants are often an indicator of more serious types of pollution to follow . Furthermore, since pollution is man-produced and the effects are suffered by man, aesthetic problems are certainly of interest. Nevertheless in any management situation when trade-offs are required, it will certainly be necessary to rank different types of pollutants so that society can determine how it would like to spend is limited funds of time, effort, and money.

Acuate Effects

Let us look first at the pathogenic pollutants since these are obviously the most important. The effects of pathogenic pollutants are either acute or chronic. Acute effects are those which occur in a relatively short period of time while chronic effects may take time to be noticed, as in the case of carcinogenic pollutants, or the effect may be noticed immediately but continued for a very long period of time. The acute effects are the easiest to determine because of the short time between administration and affection. The easiest way of measuring acute effect is by feeding the pollutant in question to test organisms, such as since or selected fish, and observing the dosage required to will 50% of the organisms involved. This is usually done by feeding a pollution of test organisms increasing amounts of the pollutant, and for each dosage the number of individuals that succumb is noted.

When these data are plotted, an S- shaped curve results, such as shown in Graph - 3.1 wherein dosage versus number of mortalities is plotted. From this curve it may be seen that there are a small number of individuals that require an extremely large does before they are killed while some are killed with a relatively small dose. By plotting this type of curve, it is easy to locate the dose for which half the individuals die. This dosage is called the LD50, and it is this LD 50 which is usually used to compare the relative toxicity of one pollutant with another.

Another way of examining acute effect is to observe the effect of a given pollutant concentration on organisms over a somewhat longer period of time, noting how long it takes for given dosage to produce mortalities. This say be done by giving a predetermined concentration of the pollutant to the test animals and observing how long it takes to kill half of them. When data from an experiment such as this are plotted, a curve similar to that shown in graph 3.2 results. As may be seen, the curve is a hyperbola with the horizontal asymptotic suggesting a threshold concentration. In other words, below this asymptotic value there is no apparent effect, since at this concentration an finite amount of time is required for mortality.

The vertical asymptote, on the other hand, appears to be a saturation level. At this level any increase in the concentration will not produce any further decrease in the amount of time required for fatality. Evidently there is a finite time required for the pathogen to do its work, so that no matter how high the concentration, the time required to kill will not go below this amount.

Charonic Effects

With the asympototic values, suggests another concept : the threshold value. There appears to be a dose size for each pathogen below which the pollutant has no effect. The concern with threshold values for various pollutants is one aspect of the study of chronic effects. Chronic effects are the most difficult to measure because of the time involved; in some cases cancers have developed as long as 25 years after initial exposure to the carcinogenic agent. Neverthless, measurements have been made and for many materials threshold value seems to describe the data reasonably well.

Most experiments need some measure of the effect on the organisms other than death, so that many different measures are used. These are : deformity in the growth of organisms, damage to particular organs, change in heartbeat or breathing rate, genetic damage to individuals, change in the rate of increase of a population, life expectancy of individuals within a particular population, and fecundity of females with the population. Unfortunately, and index may be very descriptive of the effect of a pollutant on a particular species, but it may be completely ineffective in describing what happens when this pollutant comes in contact with other species.

A typical experiment using one of these measures would involve the variation in pathogen concentration while noting the variation in the heartbeat or some other measure. When these data are plotted the result is very often a straight line as shown in graph 3.3. This linear relationship between effect and concentration may be extrapolated back to determine the concentration for zero effect. When this is done the line will cross the axis at a concentration from zero. This is called the threshold value.

A great deal of caution must be used in interpreting these data. Some pathogens apparently have no threshold value associated with them, and it is always risky business to extrapolate a straight line. The actual manner in which the organisms reacts to the stimulus might very well be nonlinear at lower dosages. In addition some chronic effects may be so suitable that two or three generations of the organisms might be required to observe any change.

Synergism

Another complication in the examination and quantification of pathogenic pollutants is the phenomenon of synergism. A synergistic effect occurs when the combined effect of two or more materials acting together is greater than would be expected from the simple sum of the individual effects. Temperature, for example, is a very strong synergistic parameter, generally enhancing most pollutant effects as temperature is increased. The same is true of salinity and dissolved oxygen. Some pollutants, on the other hand, tend to decrease the effects of others, as might be in the case of a strong acid and a strong base present at the same time. Other pollutants may cause strong pathogens to be precipitated out of the water column or to be collected on sediments, so that in either case they end up on the bottom. Thus it is extremely important in the analysis of any pollutant to be aware of the other materials present and their synergistic tendencies.

Within the marine biosphere many organisms are affected by various pollutants. Whether or not a particular organism is affected by any given pollutants will depend on any variable. For example, many polluants are found only in he water column while others, such as some of the pesticides and heavy metals, are adsorbed onto suspended sediments and usually find their way to the bottom within a relatively short period of time. Consequently, these latter types would tend to affect those organisms living on the bottom or feeding from bottom organisms more then they would affect the organisms living within the water column, such as free swimming fish.

Also of import in determining the effectiveness of a particular pollutant on living organisms is its relative solubility in water and oil. Pollutants more soluble in oil will tend to find their way to organisms that have a larger content of oil in their body issues. This is particularly true of some of the pesticides which are more soluble in oil than water. The individual habits of marine organisms also affect their susceptibility to a particular pollutant.

Feeding habits with respect to time of day, portion of water column for aged, type of material ingested, and the method of digestion utilized all determine to a great extent the types of pollutant the organism will be exposed to. Similarly spawning habits determine the type of area and time of year in which a species is particularly sensitive to subtle changes in the environment. These changes affect not only the parents but also the offspring, and may be even their progeny.

Other habits not having to do with spawning also help to determine whether an organism will be exposed to particular pollutants. Weather the organism is sensitive to light or sound, for example, will often determine whether it is attracted to a particular out-fall. Thus we find that a pure and simple cause and effect relationship between a pollutant and an organism is not enough to determine completely the actual response of the organism in the real world. Laboratory results might be completely refused in the field simply because the organism does not respond to extraneous characteristics of the environment under natural conditions in the same manner in which it did in the laboratory.

Pathways to Man

Once some of the pollutant has been ingested by marine organisms, the major concern of man is the possibility of this pollutant appearing on his dinner table and causing a pathogenic response. Obviously if a fish ingests a pollutant and a human eats that fish, then that person will have ingested a does of that pollutant and there will probably be some danger. The question is, "How much?" In order to arrive at an approximation of the actual amount of undesired material finding its wax into the reader's stomach, one mush follow the pollutant through a number of steps.

Most organisms living in the sea tend to concentrate materials existing in the sea to much greater values that they are in the ocean itself. For example, a diatom, a small form of marine algae having a silicate frustule, has a body concentration of silicon about 40 thousand times as great as the oceanic waters from which the organism derives all of its material. Thus the diatom concentrates silicon very effectively so that if we eat diatoms, a large portion of our diet would be glassy. Similarly, other organisms, including fish, will concentrate other materials even if these do not naturally occur in the environment. But this amplification or concentration does not stop with one step. We must continually keep in mind the fact that an organism does not exist by itself in the marine environment.

Any organism is dependent upon many other organisms for its existence. An edible fish, for example, might very well subsist on smaller fish which, in turn, might subsist on small zooplankton, which, in turn, may subsist on phytoplankton. There may be 5 to 10 individual links in a food chain leading to man, and there is the distinct possibility that for each one of these links a concentration of the pollutant occurs. Thus the total pathway to man for the pollutant might be a rather tortuous one, but it might result in a very high concentration of the pollutant material in the fish.

This in itself may be of no concern to the individual unless he ingests the fish and if so, how often and how much he consumes. It is not enough simply to know that there is some pollutant present in marine organisms: one also should know how much is present, and in addition two other facts are required. This first is the accepted maximum level of ingestion of the pollutant before harm results, and the second is the amount of fish that can be eaten before this level is reached. In this way it might very well be possible to have a particular kind of fish one or two times a year with perfect safety, while if it is eaten once a day, it might very well have a toxic effect.

Ecomorphic Pollutants

There are many different types of pollutants that may be classified as ecomorphic, while some pollutants fall into all three of the classes stipulated above and many fall into at least two. Sediment is a pollutant whose effect is primarily that of changing the environment since it is not pathogenic and very often is not aesthetically displeasing, although it can be. As it settles to the bottom, it will tend to bury the organisms that live on the bottom, such as oysters and clams, and eventually smother them.

Sediment also tends to fill in marsh areas, killing the marsh grass, and completely changing the habitat. Since marsh areas are breeding grounds for small fish and an important ecological link in most of the oceanic life, any destructive process such as this is bound to markedly change the marine biological environment. On the other hand, in some cases where man's activities have produced large amounts of erosion and sediment has been brought down by rivers into estuaries, some estuarine areas have been filled enough to support marsh grasses. In some cases excess erosion can produce marsh lands rather than destroy them. Whenever there is a depth change in an estuarine or coastal area, the effects are many. They range from changing the biological environment so that larger fish will no longer live in the shol areas to affecting the total circulation pattern of the area. But suffice it to say that changing depth in many cases does change the manner in which salt and fresh water mix in the coastal area and also the amount of flushing present in a particular region.

When the sediment is in suspension it also has an effect on the eco-system, the most obvious aspect being a change in transparency. By making the water more opaque, light will not penetrate as deeply as before so that the thickness of the layer of water in which plants grow will be decreased. If the water is fairly shallow to begin with, this decrease in transparency may very well result in the inability of rooted plants to grow and some marsh lands may be destroyed. The effect of sediment, then is two-fold : changing both bottom and water properties. Both of these effects tend to change the physical characteristics of the ecosystem.

Another ecomorphic pollutant is oil, although oil sometimes produces toxic effects. The result of oil coating bird feathers is a well known physical effect. The oil does not poison birds; it simply makes it impossible for them to fly and consequently many of them die. A film of oil on the surface will also decrease the amount of sunlight entering the water and, similarly, will limit the exchange of oxygen from the atmosphere. In addition to the aesthetic and pathogenic effects of oil, there are thus also ecomporphic effects.

The toxic effects of various nitrogen compounds are well known but fertilizers and other nutrients washed into the sea have a nontoxic effect on marine waters. These materials will do just what they are designed to do : make plants grow, whether these plants be terrestial or aquatic plants.

The toxic effects of various nitrogen compounds are well known but fertilizers and other nutrients washed into the sea have a nontoxic effect on marine waters. These materials will do just what they are designed to do : make plants grow, whether these plants be terrestial or aquatic plants. Those plants on the bottom of the blanket will tie, due to lack of light, and those roting plants will utilize oxygen in their decay processes. Even though there are more plants than before, producing more oxygen in the process of photosynthesis, so many of them are dying and decaying the result is to decrease the dissolved oxygen. This phenomenon is called "Eutrophication."

Another ecomorphic pollutant that seems to be receiving a lot of attention lately is heat. Usually supplied to the marine environment form electrical power plants or other industrial sources, this heat will increase the water temperature and may result in different kinds of damage to marine organisms. Since most mutations are caused to thermal activity under normal conditions, the possibility of genetic damage is real. It is estimated that about 90% of the mutations occuring normally are thermally caused, while only about 10% are caused by radiation.

Aesthetic Pollutants

The last type of pollutant mentioned above was aesthetic pollutants. Aesthetic pollutants are those which offend the human senses and as such are considered by many to be unimportant. In many environmental problem areas, though, the aesthetic considerations often receive more attention by environmentally oriented citizens than some of the pathogenic pollutants. This is simply because the aesthetic pollutants are visible and what can be seen, smelled, or heard appears much more bothersome than that which is hidden, even though the hidden pollutant might be much more dangerous to life.

Consequently, any scheme for controlling marine pollution must include some consideration of the aesthetic pollutants if it is to succeed. An excellent strategy seems to be to focus on the aesthetic pollutants and use them as a machanism to gather momentum to clean up the rest of the pollution problems.

Power transmission cable has caused more than one power company grief because of the environmental consideration given the local citizens who are concerned about the appearance of power cables running across the countryside. Oil wells, especially the offshore variety visible from resort areas, are of great concern to most environmentalists. The same thing is true of equipment required for dredging operations and the spoil areas resulting from these operations. To some people, especially those living in relatively pristine environments near the water, boats can also be an aesthetic pollutant, especially those that cause waves and noise. Effluents that cause the colour of the sea to change to increase the amount of suspended sediments also may be considered aesthetic pollutants. It simply is not as pleasant to go swimming in water that is cloudy and contains colouring material different from what one would expect in a normal, natural body of water.

In essence, any change from the pristine environment appears to many to be aesthetic pollution. Obviously we are living in an unreal world if we think the marine environment can be maintained in an unspoiled form. It should be borne in mind that many compiaints about aesthetic pollution come from individuals who would father live in the primeval environment not realizing that it would not be available to them unless the commercial world about them supported it.

There appears to be a dichotomy wherein try to maintain the unspoiled environment in certain areas while letting others become over utilized. Nevertheless, there is a growing movement to include in the cost of every project a relatively small sum to improve its aesthetic qualities. This is, of course, exactly the same philosophy that is applied to the control of other forms of pollution. Additional money is spent in a chemical process, for example, to control the pollution-producing properties of the effluent since society believes that this additional sum of money is desirable expenditure. It may similarly be maintained that the expenditure for aesthetic pollution control is desirable as it also will tend to increase the quality of life.

This paragraph briefly state those portions of these studies that are relevant to determining the effects of oil on marine wetlands. Also, the literature and out personal experiences with oiled marine wetlands are synthesized to allow an evaluation of methods or protection, cleanup, and restoration attempts that have been carried out in marine wetlands. This section accomplishes there two objectives by:

— Providing a brief review of the effects of all spills and related celanup activities on salt marshes and mangrove ecosystems

— Reviewing methods of protecting marine wetlands from being oiled.

— Reviewing successful means of cleaning marine wetlands following oil spills.

— Reviewing and presenting techniques that have proven successful in restoring marine wetlands damaged by oil spill and/or cleanup operations.

— Establishing a set of criteria and discussing guidelines for decisions on means of protecting susceptible areas, and for cleaning and restoring oiled marine wetlands.

— The differences in growth patterns and life cycles are essential elements in consideration of methods of cleanup and restoration of marine wetlands.

— It should be noted that salt marsh and mangrove vegetation occur together in some parts of the world, e.g., southern Brazil, southeast Australia. For the purpose of this discussion, we need to identify two terms.

— Recovery : return of a site to dominance by native organisms that are within the natural range of limits for structure and function in unprotected examples of the ecosystem within the local geographic area.

— Restoration: man's efforts to initiate and/or enhance the recovery process.

Effects of Oil Spills on Marshes and Mangroves

Oil impacts to marshes will vary with a number of factors including the amount of oil, type and magnitude of cleanup activities, type of oil, physical and biological structure of the marsh, latitude, and season. Subsequent persistence of damages and recovery of the system also depend on numerous physical, chemical, and biotic factors, including weathering rate and degree of removal or retention of oil, availability of propagules (seeds or vegetative), successional processes, sediment erosion/ acceration, and restrorative activities by man. Plants can be affected in several ways. Physical smothering by oil can lead to reduced transpiration, respiration, and photosynthesis.

Absorption of toxic oil fractions through the leaves or roots may cause poisoning of the plant by disrupting cell membranes and cellular organelles. Some species such as *juncusmaritimus is gerarii,* and Spartina anglica exhibit epidermal or cellular resistance to oilds. There is a considerable range of sensitivity to oil. Some species are resistant even to repeated spills (e.g., salicornea sp. Many of the more resistant species are also pernnials with large root systems that enable them to grow back following oil damage to aerial portions.

Oils vary in their toxicity, according to the content of lowboiling compounds, unsaturated compounds, and aromatics. In general, the higher the concentration of these constituents, the more toxic the oil. It is self evident that the amount of oil and frequency of oiling will effect the degree of damage, but it is less obvious that viscosity of the oil is important. With light oil, there is a physical limit to the amount that will "stick" to a shore, with subsequent tides redistributing oils. In contrast, the viscosity of heavy oils often allows retention of large volumes and many cause mortality not through toxicity but through smothering. Heavy oils also tend to be more persistent and to extend the duration of damage, thus slowing recovery.

Since and sediment structure of the marsh considerably affect the degree of damage and potentials for recovery. In the United States, Europe, and elsewhere marshes may be narrow fringing bands along the high water mark, especially in areas where tides are small, or marshes may be broad vegetational belts (occasionally many hundreds of meters wide) in estuaries or on sheltered coasts, especially where tidal ranges are large. Extensive marshes may not be completely covered even to massive spills, as oil will tend to affect the sides of the creeks and drainage channels first and then progress into the marshes plateau.

Where vegetation it tall and dense (e.g., in a spartinetum of juncetum), considerable volumes of all may be completely oiled, and after severe damage, there may be no source of propagules for recovery. In such area, restorative action may be the only means of marsh reestablishment in the short term. Sediment characteristics, including particle size distribution and drainage patterns, considerably affect potential for oil retention. Marshes in North America and Europecan be found in sediments ranging from medium grainted sands to very fine silts where more than 95% of sediment particles are less than 63 in diameter.

Sands tend to be more freely drainging and more easily penetrated by oils as shoots can occur. If oil penetrates anaerobic sediments weathering is reduced or stops, and the oil may be retained in unchanged form for considerable periods of time, reducing or preventing plant regrowth. However, where oil is weathered before or after incorporation, even very high levels may not prevent plant regrowth. Growth in solicornia sp., *suaeda maritima, Aster tripolium* and *Spartina anglica* has been reported run areas where levels of total aliphatic hydrocarbons of up to 5,875 µg/g were found. Seasonal changes in the marsh may considerably affect the extent of oil damage. Oiling before or during flowering can cause reduced flowering and seed production. This may delay flowering and seed production (Dicks, unpublished data). During winter months many species die back and oil may affect only dead and decaying vegetation; however, in spring and summer growth, new shoots and germinating seedlings are particularly vulnerable.

In some cases, a major problem following oil damage to vegetation has been loss of sediment stability followed by erosion (e.g., Isle Grande, France following the Amoco Cadiz oil spill). Where extensive rhizomatous roots mats ramify the sediments or where vegetation cover is continuous (e.g., in denise Spartina Stands), sediments may remain stable even when vegetation has been killed. In low marsh colonized mainly by annual species (e.g., Salicornica) or where vegetation is sparse, root mats may be insufficient to prevent erosion. Where erosion occurs, lowering of marsh level may prevent reestablishment of vegetation. Erosion may also follow damage to creek systems after cleanup activities (e.g., during the Amoco Cadiz spill that affected the Isle Grande marshes. The importance of slat marshes in prevention of coastline erosion is well established and may be of prime importance in some areas.

Because of the preceding considerations, basin forest may have variable characteristics. Generally, however, basin forests are well developed with canopy heights that may reach 15-20 m. Riverine forests: This forest type develops along the edges of estuaries, often as far as the inland extent of the saline intrusion. It is best developed, however, in the lower course of the estuary where water flows are moderate to high and high nutrient inputs prevail. This combination of adequate freshwater and nutrient inputs allows the development luxriant stands.

On the periphery of the forest, the dominant species is the Rhizophora mangrove. This is an area where there is greater kinetic energy by due to the combination of river flow and tidal motion. The complex root system of Rhizophora, with its extraordinarily developed adventitious ("stilt") roots, allows the establishment of large trees on very unstable, soft soild. In the inner forest, mixed stands of Laguncularia and Avicennia occur. Rieverine forests are highly productive with litter fall rates in excess of 4 g/m/day. Canopy heights reach 20 m in the best-developed forests.

Fringe forests: This type occurs along the seaward edge of forests lining protected shorelines. There is usually a strong horizontal gradient in tropography as well as a significant gradient in turbulence and tidal amplitude. Energy derived from the tides and waves decays rapidly inland where tidal flooding is further reduced by the rise in the mangrove floor. The reduced flusing inland results in the establishment of a physiochemical gradient in water quality, toward the outer edge of the fringe, where greater energy levels prevail, the large, heavy seedlings of Rhizophora become established. Inland this way and tidal energy dissipates, and in the higher, less flushed parts of the fringe, Avicennia becomes the dominant species.

Since frings are exposed, they are subjected to periodic destruction buy storms, waves, or scouring by strong current as. During storms large amounts of debris may be deposited in the outer firinge, reducing circulation to the inner firinge and the basins inland.

Overwash forests: These forests are formed on small island or projections from land masses (peninsulas) they are characterized by intense flushing by daily tides. The high flushing rates do not allow the formation of strong salinity gradients nor the accumulation and aggradation of the soil or of nutrients factors that usually lead to a succession of species toward the interior. True overwash forests are thus monospecific (cominated by rhizophora).

The amount of flushing and nutrient availability are critical factors that determine the structure and the rate of overwash forests. They, overwash islands in coastal oligotrophic waters may not be as developed as those inside coastal lagoons where higher nutrient accumulation is possible. Excessive flushing leads to erosion and loss of the forest whereas extremely low flushing rates lead to accumulation of debris and vertical aggradation inside the forest with reduced flushing rates toward the core of the island. These islands thus evolve into firings and basin forests. Cintron *et al.* have described the formation, ageing, and decay of these island in southwest Puerto Rico.

Dwarf forests : Dwarf forest are found in marginal environments where their structural development is limited by edaphic factors, probably the unavailability of nutrients, Mature trees in these forests are usually less than 3 m tall. Salinity is not the limiting factor. Although the vegetation is limited in high, leaf size is not reduced as usually happens when mangroves are under the influence of a chronic stresson. This type of forest is different from those that may be considered scrub forests and that develop under the influence of chronic stressor, such as high salinity or cold stress. The dominant species in Dwarf forest in Florida and Puerto Rico is Rhizophora.

Table 1. List 14 oil spills. Worldwide, where some documentation of impact to mangroves has been observed and reported. Most of the earlier reports are anecdotal with little or no quantification as to the levels of oil contamination; the actual types of oil stranded in the forests; the areal extent of mangroves oiled, and actual numbers, sizes, or areal coverage of magroves killed or stressed by the oil spill. In addition, the species of mangroves involved was often not mentioned. In addition to impacts to the trees themselves, the final component of the ecosystem is usually treated by noting dead or stressed animals at the time of the spill, or attempting to quantify losses or changes by one-shot sampling. In particular, the sampling of infauna, in many of these cases, has not taken into account the normal seasonal variations in infaunal species and numbers. All these problems may lead to widely different observations of the "impact" of a spill by different investigators.

Due to the fact that floating oil is transported by waves and currents and strands on shorelines, low-wave energy ecosystems such as mangroves forests are routinely sites where oil accumulates after a spill. In addition, the inaccessibility of most mangrove forests makes oil removal very difficult, if not impossible, and the fine-grained and peaty anaerobic sediments characteristic of mangrove forests may reduce the rate of microbial breakdown of oil. These factors, plus the burrowing activities of crustaceans characteristic of mangrove forests, can lead to persistent, high levels of oil contamination not only on the soil's surface but also deep in the sediments in the mangrove root core, and mangroves can be killed.

6 Cigarettes and Smoking

So far over a thousand different chemical substances have been identified in cigarette smoke. A large number of them take the form of fine dust particles which, laden with cancer forming hydrocarbons, penetrate the inner recesses of the lungs, the alveoli. One of the best-known poisons is the paralyzant nicotine. This can cause spasms and paralyze the breathing center in the brain. If present in a quantity of 50 mg it can prove fatal. One-hundredth part of this quantity (which corresponds to the amount absorbed from tobacco smoke) is enough to change the metabolism of the nerve cells perceptibly. Nicotine infiltrates from the inhaled air contaminated with cigarette smoke, into the bloodstream and irritates the autonomic nervous system. This in turn affects the heart, the stomach, and other autonomic reactions of the body. In addition to the coronary vascular system, the other arteries in the body are also damaged by nicotine.

On the average the arteries of a man who has smoked 20 cigarettes a day for 30 years can be as stiff and fragile by the time he is 50 as those of a nonsmoker fully 15 years older. As a result, circulatory disturbances and heart infarctions, strokes and other consequences of insufficient blood supply are similary more frequent. The likelihood of death from a heart infarction is 3 to 5 times greater for smokers than for nonsmokers.

The injury potential of tobacco tar in cigarette smoke has so far been researched the least. Just a few puffs from a cigarette are sufficient to arrest the self-purification mecahnism of the lungs, the minute filter hairs on the mucous membranes of the respiratory tract. The result of this for the regular smoker is a racking smoker's cough and chronic bronchitis. The tar contains a large number of poisons, which in some causes have not yet been closely analyzed.

The fine dividing walls between the alveoli in the lungs can be broken down and demolished by such poisons, and this will result in under-functioning of the lungs (emphysema), with shortage of breath and increased susceptibility to disease. In recent years the cigarette industry has turned its attention to brands containing less nicotine and tar. To judge by the results of tests conducted on animals, these milder brands of cigarettes are likely to reduce the danger of contracting bronchilal cancer from cigarette smoking. On the other hand, according to medical authorities on smoking and health, there is also a fear that additional substances contained in the milder cigarettes, such as sodium nitrate, could form new cancer-inducing substances such as nitrosamines, which are capable in certain circumstances of causing cancerous affection in other parts of the human body.

Apart from the smoker himself, the problem of the absorption of contaminants from tobacco smoke also concerns the nonsmoking "co-smoker". It is now suspected that the additional smoke from a cigarette (that which is not inhaled by the smoker), to which the co-smoker is mainly exposed, contains as many cancer-producing and other dangerous substances (nicotine, pyridine, phenols and ammonia) as the mainstream of smoke inhaled by the smoker himself. The incidental flow of smoke contains, for example, three times more cancer producing 3-4 benzopyrene than the mainstream. In the interval between puffs, all the poisonous constituents pass into the secondary flow. Members of the catering trade, such as waiters, even when they are nonsmokers, are affected more often by bronchial cancer than the rest of the population. Investigations show that cancer-producing 3, 4-benzopyrene is present in smoke-filled catering establishments in concentrations of 2.8 to 14.4 mg per cu m (compared with an average in big city atmospheres of from 0.28 to 0.48 mg per cu m).

A special danger in the matter of passive smoking occurs for the embryo of a mother who smokes during pregnancy, for there is no possibility open to the embryo of escaping from the danger zone. The number of premature and stillbirths is higher for expectant mothers who smoke than for those who do not. The weight of the baby at birth is also lower, and its subsequent mental development may be impaired.

A clinical handicap caused by co-smoking that is difficult to the assess is reduction in mental capacity. Cigarette smoke contains the poison gas carbon monoxide, which has a 250-times-higher capacity to combine with the red blood cell pigment hemoglobin that has atmospheric oxygen. The hemoglobin is obstructed thereby, is unable to absorb more oxygen, and is handicapped in performing the vital function of transmitting oxygen.

A lack of oxygen has serious consequences for the brain and the nervous system in particular. Although the brain accounts for only about 2% of the entire body weight. It requires some 2% of the oxygen intake of the body as a whole. Under these circumstances it is understandable that the finer brain functions, such as powers of concentration, decision-making, discernment and responsiveness, should be affected adversely by reduced supplies of oxygen. From a broad-based series of investigations it has emerged that non-smokers who are obliged to smoke passively are subject to the following complaints; conjunctivitis, headaches, nausea, vertigo, reduced powers of concentration, etc. Medical authorities on smoking and health and other organizations are accordingly demanding that the right of the nonsmoker to physical protection should be given priority over the smoker's right to indulge his addiction.

7 MAN-ENVIRONMENT RELATIONSHIP

The molecular oxygen supply in the atmosphere and the broad expanse of open ocean are not threatened by man's activities in the foreseeable future. Molecular oxygen is one resource that is virtually unlimited. Broecker feels that man's existence will be threatened by other types of environmental pollution long before his oxygen supply becomes endangered, and that we need not worry about total oxygen supply. This is typical of some of the different opinions which are unfolding between physical and biological scientists. Such differences often indicate the need for more research and better knowledge before we can fully accept one position on another.

Another atmospheric problem of long-term concern is the increase in carbon dioxide in the atmosphere. Between 1860 and 1960 the combustion of fuel increased the CO_2 content of the air by 14 percent of its formerly stable level, Carbon dioxide tends to reflect infrared rays from the earth, and this provides a "greenhouse effect" for the whole earth; that is, it accumulates heat. This will gradually increase the temperature of the earth—an effect which may have long-term implications in climate modification. A rise of just 2 or 3 degrees in annual mean temperature would have a major melting effect on glaciers and ice caps, and this could raise the level of the seas several feet. Such a rise in the seal level would inundate many of the world's major cities. Some experts predict it may re quire 4,000 years, and others feel it will not happen at all. The latter believe that any occurrence of the greenhouse effect due to increasing CO_2 in the atmosphere will be offset by increasing particulate pollution in the air and a cooling of the earth's surface. Once gain, we see fundamental controversies on major issues-largely because we do not really have the complete answer. The atmospheric problem may also become acute in terms of various toxic elements released into surface, air and water: carbon monoxide, sulfur dioxide, lead from automobile exhaust, hydrocarbons from industrial operations and numerous other products of modern technological societies. For example, 500 million pounds of lead are discharged into the atmosphere of the United States each year from automobile exhausts alone, and significant amounts of this become incorporated into living organisms.

A recent study in Sweden showed concentrations of lead in mosses to be as high as 300 to 500 ppm along roadsides. Some roadside plants in the United States may have lead levels up to 3,000 ppm,. This lead enters the plants via both air and water and can then enter man and animals. A hundred years ago, before the automobile, concentrations in roadside plants were less than 20 ppm. Lead levels over 0.5 ppm have detectable physiological effects in man and animals, and 1.0 ppm levels are often toxic.

In conclusion, there seems to be little or no immediate threat that we will run out of air for breathing, but several warnings have appeared regarding the quality of our air. We apparently have an adequate supply of total oxygen for many centuries to come though even this is a debatable point. In some localities the situation may be critical at certain times. If stationary inversions of air trap the polluted atmosphere over some of our largest cities such as Tokyo, London, New York or Los Angels, toxic air pollutants increase to dangerous levels. In August of 1969, a massive still-air inversion occurred in eastern United States, causing serious air pollution in urban areas from New Orleans and St. Louis, north to Chicago and Milwaukee, and east to Washington and Baltimore. At no time was there an absolute shortage of oxygen, but dangerous level of carbon monoxide, sulfur dioxide, hydrocarbons and other air pollutants accumulated in several cities.

Twenty million people were affected by varying degrees of eye irritation and respiratory diseases. Fortunately, this great blanket of smog was dispersed by upper air currents in the first week of September, and no large-scale health tragedies occurred. More serious event of this type are likely to occur in urban areas unless strong measures against air pollution are undertaken.

Worldwide water supplies represent a concern for the future of man in terms of both the quality and absolute quantity of fresh water. Many cities have reached or are coming close to their total available fresh water supply and are reaching further and further to obtain new supplies. Los Angeles, for example, is planning tremendous canals and canduits which will bring water from the pacific northwest over 1,000 miles to the growing megalopolis of southern California.

Two Russian geographers and hydrologists, Kalinin and Bykov, have pointed out that "The world's water resources from a single entity. The basic hydrologic cycle of the world depends upon solar energy, atmospheric circulation, heat reflectivity and surface retention. The latter is strongly influenced by the biotic community, kalinin and Bykov point out, on the assumption that the moisture content of the earth remains constant that the total gains and losses from the land and the sea are in balance. Thus, the total precipitation equals the total evaporative loss from land and sea. However, the relative retention time and thus the total amount of water in terrestrial and fresh-water environments can change substantially in relation to the biota and terrestrial storage capacity. A large proportion of the world's fresh water, falls and resides in relatively unpopulated portions of the globe, particularly Siberia and northern Canada. Here, man's activities are limited by other factors and he cannot readily obtain these vast stores of water.

Secondly, the matter of water quality is of immediate concern. The principle of water reuse is now becoming accepted, so that people recognize much of their water has been used previously by other municipal systems. Each reuse cycle however, is increasingly costly in terms of treatment, and each reuse cycle requires disinfectants and other industrial chemicals, combining these problems of distribution and quality, it seems that the water problem of the future is not going to be one of a global water shortage on a planetary basis but one of local crises due to the concentrations of people, industry and water use. Certainly, the immediate concern is finding local water resources of adequate quality to meet the burgeoning needs of urban populations. To the city dweller in New York or Hong Kong whose water tap runs dry or to the refugee in the Middle East who is dying of thirst, it well be little comfort to realise that 29,000,000 cubic kilometers of fresh water are locked in glaciers and polar ice caps.

World Food Supplies

Nowhere is scientific controversy more evident than on the issue of world food supplies. Some scientists predict famines and mass starvation within the next 10 years. They feel the stage is irrevocably set for millions of people to die of starvation in the 1980's. In fact, we already have famine in many parts of the world, if one defines famine as people dying of lack of food. Even at the height of the Green Revolution in Asia in which new strains of rice and wheat were producing phenomenally large yields, famine conditions existed in parts of Rajasthan in India: in sections of Burma and in southern Thailand. Starvation is now a grim reality in much of the world and it may well get worse despite the Green revolution.

Other scientists refute the pessimism and find evidence for a hopeful outlook in the world food situation. They feel that the Green Revolution which was based on new strains of rice and wheat in Asia and Africa, and which produced a doubling and tripling of yields in one or two years, shows what can be done with modern agriculture. For the first time in many decades, agricultural output increased more rapidly than population growth. India began to approach self-sufficiency in food production, and the Philippines began to export rice again for the first time since 1900.

A word of caution about the Green revolution is also necessary. It is quite true that new strains of agricultural crops can sometimes dramatically increase yields, but often these new strains require more careful management, more intensive care, more water, more fertilizer and more insecticides. They may be more vulnerable to plant viruses or fungi. Although the plant geneticists try to breed in every possible disease resistance, these new strains do not have the centuries of natural selection and regional adaptation behind them as do the local strains which the villages have always used. In West Bengal and Orissa, there were reports that some of the newly introduced high-yield strains of rice were succumbing to a disease that was not affecting that old traditional strains. If this happens to a major extent, the Green Revolution could collapse and a severe blow would be dealt to the villager's faith in the agricultural scientist. Another factor in the world food picture is one of pure climatic good fortune.

Green Revolution in India was accompanied by the best monsoon seasons in over 10 years. A long series of droughts had broken is southern Asia and adequate rains fell in the right pattern. The possibility exists, therefore, that a good part of the success of the Green Revolution was due to good weather, combined with new strains and more fertilizer. This is a question that will be more adequately answered in future year to see if increasing agricultural production can be maintained in years of poor rainfall.

In India too much rain came and it fell to early. The wheat crops in northern India were magnificent in April and May just before harvesting and threshing, but heavy premature rains in many areas caused the wheat to rot before it could be threshed. Bihar had serious crop losses from flooding. Once again, this was a tragic and dramatic demonstration that even the Green Revolution remains dependent on climatic factors outside the control of man.

Through all of these arguments on how many people the world can feed, one must ask the realistic question: "Is it necessary that there always be a race between population and food production? Is it desirable to be teetering on the brink of starvation at all times? Is it the best representation of the human condition to be struggling in this manner to feed more and more people at a subsistence level?

One also has the impression in reviewing the literature on world food supplies that too much emphasis is placed on future predictions, and not enough on current conditions. We furthermore know that malnutrition exist throughout the world, even in the most advanced countries. We furthermore know that malnutrition of many kind has profound effects upon growth, development and behavior. Children growing up with malnutrition from early infancy definitely show reduced growth rates and possible retardation of physical and mental development. They furthermore show increased susceptibility to infectious disease. Thus, we return to the issue of the quality of life, and the realization that merely preventing death by starvation does not by any means insure a quality nutritional base for adequate growth and human development. It is apparent that the problem of world food supplies will continue for some time as a problem of both quantity, and quality and especially one of distribution.

Space on Earth

In 1958 Paul Sears wrote an important essay entitled, "The Inexorable Problem of Space," in which he concluded that "Our future security may depend less upon priority in exploring outer space that upon our wisdom in managing the space in which we live".

The earth's total surface is 196,940,400 square miles of which about 30 per cent or 57,230,000 square miles is land surface. Of this total land surface, approximately 5,000,000 square miles are in Antarctica deserts, and 11,000,000 square miles are in mountainous regions. Of deserts and moutains, at least one-fourth of their jano area cannot be inhabited, so this eliminates another 5,000,000 square miles of land surface for human habitation. We are left with approximately 47,000,000 square miles of land surface, at the most, for the world's population.

The world now has nearly about 6 billion people. The world population has doubled in the past 40 years and may double again in the next century, perhaps approaching stability at about 11 billion by the year 2100. By 1990, of the world's 5.3 billion people, 4.1 billion—77 percent lived in the developing world; 1.2 billion inhabited the industrialized countries. India has nearly 1/6th of the world's population. There are 257 person per sq. km. in India. In the Capital City Delhi there are 6318 person per sq. km. Thus it is to say human population is not evenly distributed. It leads to the problem of space.

As with water, air and food, it is important to distinguish between total or potential amount of any given resource on earth and that amount which is actually utilized or practically available to man, it was pointed out in the sections on water and air that the earth's total amount is apparently adequate for many years to come, but the supply in any given city may not be of sufficient quantity or quality to support the standard of living we would like. The amount of living space per person in some cities is less than 20 square feet per person. Theoretically, we could redistribute these crowded people to provide more even spacing around the world. Obviously, this cannot be done, and if it were attempted it might wreak havoc with agricultural production.

The economic and behavioral needs of man are such that he must cluster together, but in so doing, he creates superdensities such as Calcutta, London, New York, Paris, Tokyo, Shanghai and Buenos Aires. The slums of which are definitely deleterious to human health and welfare. Why, we might ask, does man insist on this degree of crowding and then complain about it so bitterly? Why do people continue to pour into the cities of the world when they are already known as centers of population crime and illness?

Perhaps we need to know more about the real spatial and social needs of man. What are his requirements for space and privacy, and how do these interact with his needs for social stimulation and group activity? Does man become conditioned to crowding in early childhood and then seek further crowding throughout his life? Does he require the social pressure of a crowd because he feels a compulsion to be in touch with the group and thus be able to predict what the group is going to do next? Have we produced, in our urban centers, self-destructive, systems which so modify the behavior of their inhabitants that these inhabitants exaggerate their own problems and can no longer achieve rational solutions? These are all tough question that cannot be answered in simple or easy terms. The answers will require the best intelligence we can muster from many disciplines. Some sorts of answers will certainly be necessary before we can even begin to solve the ecologic and behavioral problems associated with our own use of terrestrial space.

Distributional Inequality

With all of the last four life-support requirements of man-air, water, food and space—we have seen that the major problem of immediate importance lie in distribution more than in total amount. Technologist therefore look upon these problems as soluble by technological means. They feel, they are essentially matters of economics and transportation Behavioral and environmental scientists see them as more basic, however, relating to man's fundamental ecologic behavior. They feel, they are essentially matters of economics and transportation. Behavioral and environmental scientists see them as more basic, however, relating to man's fundamental ecologic behavior.

Certain basic social and ecologic tendencies of man prevent equitable distributions of the earth's resources. Obviously this type of argument can go on forever, and it is perhaps necessary to take a pragmatic approach and look at the current picture for the best glimpse of the future. Many of the industrial nations of the world, especially the United States, the national northern Europe and

Japan, have enjoyed rising prosperity for the last 25 years. In ecologic time, of course, this is but a flash in the pan, but let us assume that it can be sustained for another 25 or 50 years. It is worth examining where the material and energetic support for this prosperity arises. This distributional inequality is another major symptom of ecologic instability in the world. One would hope for some narrowing in the gap between the haves and the have-nots, but unfortunately the opposite trend is still occurring.

The wealthy nations of the world are far outstripping the poor nations in their rates of economic gain and human betterment. There are, however, self-corrective mechanisms within this system as, for example, when some segment of the labour it can find which will do a satisfactory job. Thus, there has been a great expansion of manufacturing in Japan, Hong Kong, Taiwan and Singapore in industries as diverse as steel, electronics, textiles, toys and optics. The Western factory worker experiences for the first time an improving situation. The western industrial worker continues to refuse his own working prospects by striking for higher and higher wages. This will certainly be one mechanism by which wealth is more adequately balanced between nations.

Still the mass of poverty throughout much of Asia, Africa and Latin America is so great that it is difficult to imagine a painless equilibrium. The differential distribution of wealth remains sharp and represents a type of ecologic situation which cannot last indefinitely without severe consequences and reverberations. To the ecologist it means either a successional stage which is not yet mature, or a system headed for a major breakdown. Economic and ecologic maturity should ideally be in the direction of broader and more equitable distribution of the earth's resources—a narrowing of the gap between the haves and the have-nots, both within and between nations, provided the total system does not pass beyond the state of corrective change.

Violence and War

Any ecological system or biotic community can be overloaded to the point of collapse by a variety of factors. Certainly one of the factors for man of most immediate and realistic danger is that of social violence. Either by war or by civil riot, man threatens his own existence.

To maintain a sense of physical security man has built an incredible stockpile of destructive power. The nations of the world spend more than 200 billion dollars per year on armaments—more than on health education, welfare, agriculture, child care and care for the aged combined. Twenty tons of explosives are stored in the world for every man, women and child. Russia and the United States have stockpiled 6,000 nuclear war heads possessing thousands of megatons of explosive force. Each megaton has more destructive power than which existed in any of the previous wars of history.

The world spends almost 8,000 dollars per year training each soldier and less than 100 dollars per year educating each child. The question is, of course, how long can man continue to preside over armament like this without using it? And the answer seems to be, not very long. The fact is we do use part of the power in an attempt to achieve social goals. It is being used daily in various parts of the world to maintain territory and dominance ranks. It is justified as a spare and deliberate use in hopes of avoiding the all out effort. How long this can continue is anyone's guess, and the ecologist can claim no more omniscience than the political scientist. The ecologist points out, however, that the ecologic and social pressures which generate international military tension may rise with increased population pressure. It is not likely that man can solve the problems of war and violence until he approaches and understands their basic orgins in terms of the behavioral and ecologic relationship between social groups, and the environment.

Adaptive Capabilities of Man

Many scholars feel that one of the great problems of the present and the future is the rapid rate of change which is occurring in society and technology. There is not, however, agreement on the consequences of the rapid change, changing life patterns are too rapid for man to adapt successfully.

Mankind is so overstimulated by the increase in new sight and sounds, so bombarded by world wide mass media, and so constantly beset with noval situations and new problems that he will break down psychologically and physically. His responses will be maladaptive and pathologic. He will thus collapse under sensory overload. It is quite possible that each of these points of view has large elements of truth in it. In the present world one can find many examples of both. Our mental institutions are already filled with those who could not adapt to sensory overload and who experience a personal breakdown of physical and mental health. Yet one can find people are living a sub-human existence where the quality of life is so low that the amount of human pain and misery seem unbearable. Yet man has adapted successfully to these inhuman conditions.

In many ways, the future is with us now. We can find throughout the world an abundance of high quality life in high quality environments, but we can also find an abundance of low quality life in impoverished environments. Many of the questions about the future revolve, therefore, around the question of relative balance and proportions. Which way are we heading and which way will the scales tip?

A major aspect of the future centers around our sense of responsibility to posterity. No representative of posterity is here to speak for the segment of society. How do the present populations of mankind regard their obligations to future generations? Are we willing to be more conservative in our life requirements, and are we, in fact, willing to reduce our rates of personal economic growth to insure a better environment and a greater abundance of resources for future generations? This may be one of the central issues of the next twenty years, and one on which the quality of present and future environments depends.

World-Wide Environmental Issues

Environmental problems have become a global issue: Some of the world wide issues are briefly described below:

(a) Climatic changes/Green house effect

Many studies show that the atmospheric pollution is on a global scale. Today, however, it is not only the air over our cities that is polluted, the entire atmosphere of our planet is now afflicted to some degree. Meteorologists talk about a nebulous veil of air pollution encircling the entire earth. Smong has been observed over the North Pole, and in their unlikely places. There are range of environmental pollution issues originating largely in developed countries which are also of global significance.

Carbon dioxide (CO_2) build-up leading to climate change is one of those key issues. Recent research indicates that increasing concentrations of CO_2 in the atmosphere, due mainly to the burning of fossil fuels could cause a warming trend leading to climate change in the next century. While there is still scientific uncertainty about the pace and impact of such a change it could be of sufficient magnitude to produce major physical, economic and social dislocations on a global scale. A special challenge posed by the issue is that if preventive actions are postponed until some effects are perceived, it may be too late to avoid appreciable climate change. It is therefore in the interests of all nations to support international efforts to understand the phenomenon at early enough stage for action to be taken to reduce or avoid major economic, social and environmental disruptions around the world. However, as developed countries are currently responsible for over two thirds of total world emissions of CO_2 by fossil fuel combustion, they have a special responsibility for supporting and contributing to accelerated efforts to assess more precisely the nature of the problems and the alternatives for action to reduce or avoid any serious risks.

Another issue is the world-wide distribution and use of harmful or potentially harmful chemicals. There are now some 70,000 chemicals on the commercial market, and many are currently used and released into the environment with little or no knowledge of their potential long-term effects. It is estimated that another 1,000 new chemicals enter the market each year. Chemicals cross national boundaries in a variety of ways: they are transported by winds and water.

(b) Risks to Ozone Layer

Ozone is a different form of life sustaining oxygen, having three atoms instead of the usual two. But this third atom, scientists have found, is very unstable and can be eliminated by chlorine ions.

The scientist have now found a close link between the family foam mattress, refrigerator and the air conditioning system of an average home and Ozone layer, 50 to 70 kilometers above the earth. They believe that free chlorine ions into the atmosphere, from plastics and other chemicals remove that extra atom of oxygen which makes Ozone. Only, in this case, the loss of the one atom changes the ability of the layer to act as a strainer to absorb the damaging ultraviolet B wavelengths from the sunlight. The findings by the experts have revealed that the rate of Ozone Layer depletion is sufficiently large to present serious consequences for man, animals and plants. In addition, new threats to the ozone layer are being recognized.

Take, for example, the refrigeration industry. Food preservation has become a necessity and refrigeration is here to stay. Only advanced technology can provide the solution to prevent the release of the damaging ions. Another example is nitrogenous fertilizer which, it is suspected, release chemicals damaging to the Ozone layer. The demand for more food and the booming green revolution in many developing countries have pushed up the use of this fertilizer. Today the world uses about 50 megatons of it. In another 20 years the rate of uses will be 100-200 megatons.

Though the Ozone Layer accounts for less than one millionth part of the earth's atmosphere, it is of vital importance to the earth's life form. It has two main functions: first it absorbs the UV-B while allowing the heat generating infra-red rays to reach the earth freely. The heat from infrared rays sustains plants and human lives by keeping the temperature of the planet at a desired level. Secondly, it influences the whether by stabilizing the stratosphere which acts as a cap to the turbulent weather system in the troposphere.

Scientists knowledge of the Ozone layer is still limited for want of advanced technology. The presence of other substances in the stratosphere, which absorbs UV-B, makes it difficult to come to a numerical and logical conclusion. But the scientists do agree that an average 70 per cent of the total UV-B reaching this planet falls on the equatorial regions between the latitudes 30° S and 30° N. They also agree that for genetic reasons people with light eyes and light skin (including albinos) are most affected by UV-B. Scientists today claim UV-B can destroy micro-organisms outright as well as cells in plants and animals. It also destroys the DN molecules and the genetic cell composition. Under natural conditions plants and animals have developed behavioural adaptation but gradual or sudden increase in UV radiation due to changes in the Ozone Layer is likely to disturb this balance.

While the scientists agree that UV-B contributes to the induction of cancer they agree the dose response relationships are too complex and unknown. These make the quantitative analysis speculative, as regards the cause of melanoma cancer and resulting deaths.

The North European Conference of Scientists November, 1980, warned that non-melanoma skin cancer in light-skinned people would increase and many crops and many acquatic organisms, including shrimps ad fish eggs, could be damaged by increased UV-B infiltration. This could even affect the reproductive process of plants and animals. It recommended that existing satellite and ground based ozone observing system should be integrated through Global Ozone Observing System (GOOS). They also recommended updating of equipment and setting up of more stations for observing the ozone system.

The scientists concerned with outer limits of the biosphere felt they are not yet technically equipped to measure accurately the rate of ozone depletion-already depleted by one percent. Though the danger is known, science has not yet provided a perfect model of measuring the depletion rate.

(c) Acid Rain

Every one realises how important the rain is. Without it the continents would be barren. Yet now the rain in parts of the earth has taken on a new and threatening complexity. It mixes in the air with pollution from burning fossil fuels particularly in power stations, factories and motor vehicles and brings down dilute sulphuric acid. This is killing fish and water life, and corroding buildings, including some of the world's most important ancient monuments. It may also damage forest and croplands, and possibly pose a substantial threat to health.

Acid rain is now recognized as an international problem. The air of industrial towns partly is cleared by chimneys at factories which push the pollution high into the air. These chimneys have made the things better locally by dispersing the pollutants, but aggravated the international difficulties. For the sulphur and nitrogen compounds emitted by burning fossil fuels can be blown thousands of kilometers by the winds, to cause acid rain in countries far from their points of origin. A special conference on acidification of the environment was held in Stockholm in 1982. It reviewed and assessed a large amount of scientific information not previously available.

So far, acid rain has been seen as an essentially regional problem, confined to the industrial areas of the northern hemisphere. But, though the problem was first perceived there, it may become much more widespread for acid rain is likely to occur wherever fossil fuels are intensively used.

Acidification is an environmental problem, or becoming one, in parts of Europe and North America. Similarly polluted areas are likely to exist elsewhere in the world, especially around large urban and industrial coagulumerations. Soils are normally much better able to resist acidification than lakes, rivers and streams. Meanwhile, acid accelerates corrosion in most materials used in construction of historic buildings, and other important cultural objects. Some of th worlds greatest cultural treasures including Parthenon in Athens and Trojans' column in Rome are being eaten away by acid fall out. There must be more effort to research and develop ways of improving energy conservation, environmentally appropriate technologies for producing heat and power, and techniques for removing sulphur from fossil fuels and gaseous emissions.

The problem of acidification may well spread to new areas as a result of rapid industrialization and the growth of cities in other parts of the world, particularly developing countries. So it is important that areas affected by acid deposition and susceptible to damage from acidification are identified as soon as possible. It they are, the damage could be mitigated or even avoided of a minimum cost to society by initiating research and applying what we already know about pollution control.

(d) Pollution of World's Oceans

The data collected from the Baltic, the North Sea, and some North American and Australian stuaries and coastal waters suggest that in most of these areas the pollution that caused most concern was due to sewage, agricultural chemicals, oil and metals.

Metal concentrations were clearly elevated in coastal waters, and in fish and shelfish living there. In some areas, mercury levels in species such as tuna were high enough to make these fish unsuitable as human food, (Perhaps the most notorious incident of all is the outbreak of "Minamata Disease" in Japan. Methylmercury discharged from a chemical factory into the sea, or produced in the sea from inorgnic mercury discharges, contaminated the fish eaten by local people at the town of Minamata of Kyushu island, Japan. As a result of this and a similar incident at Nilgata on the east coast of Honshu, nearly two thousand people have so far suffered neurological disorders; about four hundred have died).

Some of the pollution came via river; the amount of iron, manganese, copper, zinc, lead, tin and antimony that reached the sea by this route was far greater than would be supplied by natural geological processes. Other contaminants came through atmospheric deposition: the importance of this pathway for metals and synthetic chemicals was increasingly recognized during the decade (1972-82). Offshore oil and gas exploration and dredging for sand and gravel in coastal areas increased during the period 1972-1982. Coastal zone development affected extensive estuarine areas, as well as mangrove swamps and coral reefs. Oil pollution killed sea-birds fouled beaches and affected tourism. Although tanker accidents were the source of less than 5 percent of all the oil entering the sea, accidents released large volumes in small areas, and were therefore especially damaging.

A recent report issued by a group of experts on marine pollution and published by the United Nations Environmental Programme, Warns that increasing contamination of the coastal seas, which has so far only caused localized disturbances to the marine environment may become much more serious. The combined effects of the dumping of sewage sludge industrial wastes, litter and oil spills into the Mediterranean, the North Sea, the Baltic and the Gulf of Mexico, may well cause ecological disasters which could gradually lead to a global crisis since the oceans are a unified life support system. The report points out that the sea's capacity to absorb wastes has its limits, so that as the world economy continues to grow, even more sewage, industrial wastes and other effluents are likely to find their way into the sea.

Man-made radioactive materials have been discovered in the open ocean and scientists have found traces of DDT in th Arctic sea and the Antarctic penguin, thousands of miles away from the areas where the pesticide is used. And because many of the disturbances which are introduced occur at vulnerable points such as the surface of the sea or on the sea floor, where oceanic life-supporting processes are generated, the dangers and magnified.

Although the modification of this microlayer has occurred only on the vicinity of oil spills and around the marine dump site of municipal wastes and no evidence has yet been found that detergents in the open ocean have significantly influenced the properties of the sea surface, the report points out that environmental catastrophies in certain coastal areas and seas might already have occurred. Only improved management of the coastal areas and seas which involves controlling more closely the dumping of pollutants and careful monitoring of contaminant levels, will prevent a further deterioration of coastal environments. Much work however is still to be done before the several ecological sub-systems which constitute the ocean are fully understood. By the end of 1982 action plans were in operation or planned for 10 regions involving some 100 coastal States. Coastal and marine national parks and reserves were extended.

(e) Desertification

Desertification is now perceived as an intensifing world wide threat which, to varying degress, affects over 100 Member States of the United Nations. More than 20 percent of the world's population (850 million people) live in the 35 percent of the Earth's land surface (45 million km) which consists of the arid, semi-arid and sub-humid zones which is at risk of desertification. Three quarters of this area is already at least moderately desertified. Each year an additional 21 million hectares of agricultural land deteriorates through desertification to a point at which it is no longer economically productive. The last production has been valued at 26 billion dollars annually. Although desertfication is exacerbate by severe drought, its principal cause is human over exploitation of dry lands through over-cultivation, overgrazing, poor irrigation practices and deforestation. When drought strikes the overtaxed livelihood systems, desertification results.

The most devastating environmental and economic effects of desertification are in developing countries in the drylands. National balance of payments problems and local rural poverty lead to over-exploitation of lands and forests for food, fuel, cash crops and meat for export. As these and other pressures increase to unsustainable levels, agricultural productivity and soil fertility decline, creating in turn new pressures which lead to further degradation. Recovery of land for agricultural purposes become costly and often economically unfeasible, thereby reducing the economic potential of the affected countries. In many of these countries agricultural land is also being reduced by salinization, urban sprawl and sand-dune encroachment.

Increased desertification in one part of the world can indirectly induce desertification else where, as loss of agricultural land and increased food demand raise Prices and intensify pressures on marginal drylands in other food exporting and importing countries alike. There are also other impacts on international trade, to the extent that developing countries affected by rapid desertification will have a reduced capacity to import goods and services from developed countries and from other developing countries. Other globally shared impacts include loss of valuable genetic resources, disruption of hydrological cycles and increase of atmospheric dust.

A great deal is already known about the causes and effects of desertification and about the measures needed to halt or combat it. Moreover, there is favourable cost benefit ration to justify, preventive action. The 1980 estimate for implementing the 1977 plan of Action to combat Desertification was 2.4 billion dollar annually over 20 years, which is only a fraction of the estimated value of agricultural production lost each year through desertification.

It is, therefore, in the interests of all countries to establish some concreate cooperative actions between groups of developed and developing countries to halt further desertification, a goal which can be achieved, given a sufficient allocation of resources, on the basis of currently available knowledge.

(f) Loss of Tropical Forests

Although tropical forests are found in early half of all United Nations Member States, most are in twenty countries and nearly half their total area in three countries alone (Brazil, Indonesia and Zaire). The tropical forests are the world's richest biological zones, and are estimated to contain as much as 40 per cent of all terrestrial species on the planet. In addition, tropical forests provide a wide range of useful products of economic significance for both developing and developed countries. Undisturbed tropical forests are also home to millions of the world's tribal peoples.

Many experts contend that tropical forests are being exploited at a rate and in a way that is ecologically destructive and economically unsustainable. There are varying estimates of how much of the tropical forests will be lost by the year 2000 through complete conversion to other uses and by severe degradation. The results of the tropical forests resources assessment project conducted by FAO and UNEP indicated an estimated minimum loss of closed tropical forests of 12.5 per cent by the year 2000 (an average of 7.5 million hectares annually between 1980-2000) through complete conversion to other uses alone. Other studies which not only consider complete conversion but also include severe degradation caused, for example, by logging operations, by over-grazing, by over-exploitation for fuelwood, or by natural causes such as fires, insects and diseases, have estimated losses of tropical forests as upto 20 million hectares or more in a year. The FAO/UNEP study estimates that tree planting on industrial and non-industrial plantations accounts for only 10 per cent of the area of tropical forests cleared annually.

The major causes of deforestation differ by region. According to the FAO/UNEP report in Latin America the two major causes are shifting cultivation and the conversion to pasture land for cattle ranching. In Asia and Africa, shifting cultivation by subsistence farmers and removals for fuelwood are major causes. The extraction of timber from tropical forests for industrial purposes is not considered by the FAO/UNEP reports as a major factor in deforestation. On a world-wide basis, the UNEP report estimates that fuelwood and charcoal removals from tropical forests are as much as eight times greater than for industrial wood.

Serious degradation of loss of watershed forests in particular has a wide range of major ecological and economic effects through increased erosion, floods, landslides, and silting of hydro-electric facilities, irrigation systems reservoirs and harbours. The lives and livelihood of half the world's population depend directly on the wise management of watershed forests and eco-systems. Deforestation also influences local, regional and possibly even global climatic conditions by altering hydrological regions, reducing vegetation cover and causing more heat and light to be reflected back to the atmosphere (the albedo effect), and through accelerated burning of the forest biomass, which contributes to carbon dioxide build-up in the atmosphere and the global warming trend.

The economic, social and political implications of possible regional and global climate changes have only begun to be assessed.

(g) Soil Loss

Almost every environmental concern connects clearly with the importance of soil. Soil acts as a reservoir for water and other inorganic substances cycling through the eco-system. It provides habitat for many of the different populations or decomposer organisms that control the rate and capacity of nutrient recycling. The importance of soil to agriculture can hardly be over emphasised. Agriculture provides about 44 percent of the poorest countries gross domestic product and 83 percent of their employment.

Growing more food, building irrigation projects, conserving nature and precious wildlife and other needs must depend on proper soil management. The wide-ranging importance of soil confirms that soil management must consequently be many-sided. The broad range of natural and man-made stress that causes the two type of soil damage: physical displacement and alterations in soild structure and composition.

Uncontrolled shifting cultivation, salinization and water-logging flooding and plant cover destruction are same. An appropriate use of chemicals, weapons testing and deployment in warfare are some other casuses of soil nutrients and other types of soil degradation. Soil damage is also caused by patterns of dry land mountain side cultivation that carried out without arrangements for bunding and terracing to protect the topsoil.

Continuous cropping to meet growing food needs leave title time for soil conservation techniques. Deterioration of the productive capacity of the soil is most acute in areas affected by erosion, drought, mineral stress and other related factors. Soil resources that are vulnerable to these factors constitute 82 percent lands in South Asia.

While erosion is an integral part of the natural system, occurring even when land is covered by grass, or trees, its extent and intensity can be minimized provided land denudation is correspondingly reduced. The fact that it takes nature 100 years or more to build one inch of top soil should have engineered the vigilant observance of soil conservation measures. Instead, problems of soil erosion have continued ticking. Countries in East and South Asia are particularly burdened with soil erosion occuring in watersheds.

Anticipated acceleration of agricultural production and other activities between now and 2000 is casting its shadows: existing cultivable land will be further subjected to intensified use as cultivation of unsuitable areas persists; logging, firewood gathering and grazing will accelerate the elimination of vegetative cover, while the construction of roads, mine and water resources projects will be further pursued in the course of development. Such prospects place the least developed countries in an even more precarious situation.

Slash and burn farming is a common enough culprit. Wielding destruction in gradual succession, it initially causes the loss of fertility by the thin topsoil, and later eroding its stability. In India, slash and burn farming is particularly rampant in the north-eastern and central regions affecting between six and eight million hectares of land.

Salinization affects 80 million hectares (8 percent) of total land in South Asia. Something should also be said about agricultural techniques which are designed to raise land productivity but instead lead to soil loss. The use of cheap nitrogen, for example, replaces nitrogens, fixing legumes, resulting in loss to topsoil. The commonality of problems, in addition to the implications transboundary soil management points up to the fact that soil problems cannot always be resolved within the context or national concerns. Clearly, what are required are mutual policies and strategies concerning land management, and the World Soils Policy provides an appropriate starting point.

Working in collaboration with the relevant UN bodies, UNEP has proposed the World soils Policy programme which endeavours to enhance international awareness, assist countries in the formulation of national soil policies, help develop technical and scientific knowledge and collect, compile and disseminate data on the use and management of the worlds soil resources.

(h) Depletion of genetic resources

25,000 species and more than 1,000 vertebrate species and sub-species are now estimated to be threatened with extinction, yet these two categories of organisms represent only a small proportion of the terrestrial species on the planet. According to some estimates as much as from half a million to a million species would be extinguished over the next two decades. Extinction of species on this compressed scale would be without precedent in human history.

As much as two-thirds of all terrestrial species and the majority of endoangered species are located in developing countries. A significant loss of species in developing countries would have a world wide effect on future agriculture, industry and science, and on human health and welfare generally. The most serious threat to many species is the disruption and destruction of their habitat by man, especially in the tropical forests which alone harbour as much as 40 per cent of all terrestrial species. Significant species loss could directly affect human health and welfare locally, and even nationally, in many developing countries, where wild plants and animals are a source of fodder, traditional medicines and income especially for the poor in rural areas. In some countries tourism largely on wildlife is a major source of foreign exchange. In many developed countries over one-thrid of the gain in the productivity of many major agricultural crops over the last few decades has been attributed to breeding programmes using genetic material from related wild plant varieties, many of which are found in developing countries.

Moreover, many of the major crops in developed countries now have a limited genetic base. For example, more than half the Canadian prairie wheatlands are devoted to a single variety, Neepawa, which was developed with germplasm from Kenya; 72 per cent of United states potato production depends on only four varieties; and the entire United States soyabean industry is derived from a mere six plants from Asia. A significant loss of relavant wild species could limit the possibilities for maintaining or increasing the yields of major crops, such a wheat, maize, rice potatoes and for combating new strains of diseases or pests which threaten them.

Genetic stocks from one part of the world frequently make an enormous contribution to another. Current research shows that enormous opportunities lie ahead, such as the utilization of Asian blue-green algae of fix nitrogen for crop fertilization, which may constitute a gain of hundreds of millions of dolars a year to the economics of developed countries alone.

Major medicines and other pharmaceutical products in developed countries are also often dependent on plant and animal species. For the United States of America it has been estimated that more than 40 per cent of the prescriptions written each year contain a drug of natural origin-from higher plants (25 per cent), microbes (13 per cent) or animals (3 per cent) as the sole active ingredient or as one of the main ones. It has been estimated that among the 10 percent of species that might be extinguished by the year 2000 there could be many plants with potential for use in new plantbased drugs and pharmaceuticals with a combined world wide commercial sales value of as much as 200 million pounds annually.

Biomedical research in developed countries is also vitally dependent on wild species, many of which are threatend with extinction. The innovative capacity and future of the rapidly expanding field of bio-technology, practised largely in developed countries, relies considerably on genetic patterns and resources from many wild plants and animals as only about 10 per cent of the world's plant species and 1 per cent of the animal, species have so far been subjected to even a preliminary screening for potential medical or commercial applications, a significant loss of species could also represent a permanent loss of sources for more effective chemicals, medicines and other useful products.

In spite of this interdependent relationship, species loss continues to accelerate. Developing countries often lack the capacity and economic incentive for extensive species protection. They have derived little or no economic benefit from the development and use of genetic materials in developed countries, where the scientific and technical expertise to exploit species and their genetic resources predominantly resides. Nevertheless, developing countries are and will remain the principal source of genetic materials from wild plants and animals. This clearly shows that there is a common incentive for developed and developing nations to prevent a potentially catastrophic loss of species.

The mutual advantage of comprehensive joint effort could result in new medicines and other useful products that would contribute to improved levels of human health and welfare in all countries.

New Approaches to Environment and Development

Human progress has always depended on our technical ingenuity and a capacity for cooperative action. These qualities have often been used constructively to achieve development and environmental progress: in air and water pollution control, for example, and in increasing the efficiency of material and energy use. Many countries have increased food production and reduced population growth rates. Some technological advances, particularly in medicine, have been widely shared. But this is not enough. Failures to manage the environment and to sustain development threaten to overwhelm all countries.

Environment and development are not separate challenges: they are inexorably linked. Development cannot subsist upon a deteriorating environmental resource base: the environment cannot be protected when growth leaves out of account the costs of environmental destruction. These problems cannot be treated separately by fragmented institutions and policies. They are linked in a complex system of cause and effect.

First, environmental stresses are linked one to another. For example, deforestation by increasing run off, accelerates soil erosion and siltation of rivers and lakes. Air pollution and acidification play their part in killing forests and lakes. Such links mean that several different problems must be tackled simultaneously. And success in one area, such as forest protection, can improve chances of success in another ares, such as soil conservation.

Second, environmental stresses and patterns of economic development are linked one to another. Thus agricultural policies may lie at the root of land, water, and forest degradation. Energy policies are associated with the global greenhouse effect, with acidification, and with deforestation for fuelwood in many developing nations. At these stresses all threaten economic development. Thus economics and ecology must be completely integrated in decision-making and law making processes not just to protect the environment, but also to protect and promote development. Economy is not just about the production of wealth, and ecology is not just about the protection of nature: they are both equally relevant for improving the lot of humankind.

Third, environmental and economic problems are linked to many social and political factors. For example, the rapid population growth that has so profound an impact on the environment and on development in may regions is driven partly by such factors as the status of women in society and other cultural values. Also, environmental stress and uneven development can increase social tensions. It could be argued that the distribution of power and influence within society lies at the heart of most environment and development challenges. Hence new approaches must involve programmes of social development, particularly to improve the position of women in society, to protect vulnerable groups and to promote local participation in decision making.

Finally, the systemic features operate not merely within but also between nations. National boundaries have become so porous that traditional distinctions between matters of local, national, and international significance have become blurred. Ecosystems do not respect national boundaries. Water pollution moves through shared rivers, lakes, and seas. The atmosphere carries air pollution over vast distances. Major accidents—particularly those at nuclear reactors or at plants or warehouses containing toxic materials—can have widespread regional effects.

Many environment-economy links also operate globally. For instance, the highly subsidized, incentive driven agriculture of industrialized market economies generates surpluses that depress prices and erode the viability of the often neglected agriculture of developing countries. Soils and other environmental resources suffer in both systems. Each country may devise national agricultural policies to secure short-term economic and political gains, but no nation alone can devise policies to deal effectively with the financial economic, and ecological costs of the agricultural and trade policies of other nations.

8 Effects of Pesticides

The principle according to which the legal limits for pesticides are laid down require that a sufficiently large population of at least two species of animal should be thoroughly examined for at least tw.o years to establish the level (in milligrams per kilogram of body weight) at which a pesticide does no medical damage. In ordinary circumstances, one-hundredth part of this dose is then prescribed as the safe limit for a human being. Whether this security factor for human beings serves its purpose is disputed of the following reasons:

1. The applicability of the results of experiments on animals to human beings is questionable, because men are more sensitive in many essential respects than animals (e.g., in the nervous system, and with regard to the more complicated metabolism). One example of this problem is provided by the Contegran (thalidomide) catastrophe. Individual species display marked difference in sensitivity to thalidomide. While in the experimental rat, a dose of 50 mg of thalidomide per kg body weight per day was needed to produce teratogenic damage (malformation), the corresponding teratogenic dose for man was no more than 0.5-1 mg per kg.
2. For the experiments on animals, only healthy animals were used. The effect of the pesticides on

human beings afflicted by disease or other environmental influences has not been investigated.

3. Investigations into mutagenic (hereditable) effects is insufficient.
4. Only about 15% of the pesticides were examined for cancerous effects. And many of those investigated were not tested thoroughly, sometimes on only one species of animal and in limited doses.
5. Most of the substances harmful to the body are converted or decomposed in the body. But decomposition is not synonymous with detoxification. Conversion and decomposition products are in many cases more toxic than the initial product. The formation and effect of conversion products depend primarily on the specific metabolism of the individual organism chemical substances can thus display different toxic effects in different organisms.
6. In each experiment on animals, only the effect of a particular poison is tested. The possible combined effects of several poisons is thus not examined. In the case of some poisons the effects increase in geometric progression. On top of this there are combination possibilities with other environmental poisons, medicines, foodstuff additives, beverages, etc.

Traces of pesticides are detectable in about half of the samples prepared from food bought in grocery stores around the United States. About 3% of these food samples have residues that exceed the legally prescribed limits or are considered excessive. The residues most frequently found include chlorine-containing compounds, such as dieldrin and DDE (a residue of DDT), in dairy products, meat, fish and poultry, and phosphorus-containing chemicals, such as malathion, and parathion in fruits and vegetables. How much damage to human health is caused by these toxic residues? In the case of an acute toxic effect, it is normally easy to reconstruct the connection between the poison and the illness, as only a short period will elapse between the effects of the poison and the manifestation of the disease.

Acute toxic effects occur for the most part as a result of high concentration which arise in the case of pesticides only from occupational exposure, incompetent handling deliberate poisoning or accidents. Much more problematic to the general population is any chronic toxic effects caused by a gradual buildup of one or more poisons over a long period. In these cases the causal connection is hard to establish because of the time lag, the possibility of the combined effects of several toxic substances, and, in the case of pesticide residues in food, the lack of records on the type and quantity of poisons that may be involved.

One might assume that organic phosphorus compounds used as insecticides in agriculture and as insect sprays and insect strips in the home are poisonous only if taken into the body in large quantities, and that in smaller quantities they are rapidly broken down by the organism. Recent investigations show, however, that such compounds may cause long-term effects in the human body, such as cancer and hereditary damage.

The potential toxic effects of DDT, now forbidden for general use in the United States and other Western countries, have long been recognized. Patients dying from a wide variety of cause-brain tumors, brain hemorhage, high blood pressure, cirrhosis of the liver, and various forms of cancer—have been found to have a high DDT content in their fatty tissues. Virtually all animals and people in the United States carry traces of DDT and other persistent pesticide residues.

Contaminants of pesticides themselves are also suspected of having serious consequences on human health. The herbicide known as Agent Orange, used by American forces to clear vegetation in Vietnam, contained 10 to 15 ppm (parts per million) of toxic compounds called dioxin. Thus through extremely heavy spraying and dumping of Agent Orange, an estimated 1000 pounds of dioxin entered the environment. The toxic compound has been measured subsequently in South Vietnamese river fish, shellfish and human milk; and increased rates of stillbirths and births of deformed babies have been reported by both the South Vietnamese and those American families whose husbands served in the area during the Vietnam War.

Pesticides also can be converted into chemicals potentially more dangerous than the original form. The insecticide heptachlor is converted by sunlight into a stable substance some 22 times as toxic as the original substance. Once it gets into the environment, this transformation product, which like DDT is decomposed again only with great difficulty, is considerably more toxic than DDT. Many pesticides have the unfortunate quality of concentrating in the food chain. High concentrations of various pesticide residues have thus been found in mother's milk. One example is benzene hexachloride (lindane), an insecticide used in in agriculture as seed dressing. Benzene hexachloride can be so concentrated in mother's milk that in some cases the milk is contaminated 10 times more severely than is permissible for cows' milk. DDT residues are also frequently found in human milk.

Recently it has been recognized that some pesticides in very low concentrations can produce neuropsychic variations in man, such as poor concentration, troubled sleep, nausea, increased aggressiveness, and impaired muscle control. So far only a few pesticides have been examined in this respect.

As pesticides are destructive of life, on dissemination in the environment they can cause severe ecological changes. One of the most important changes relates to the powers of resistance built up in the pests affected: living organisms have the capacity to build up defense mechanisms and to develop strains that are resistant to particular poisons. By reason of mutations caused by natural or artificial substances, individual specimens constantly crop up in which a particular quality is changed in relation to the parents. Such a quality could be the capacity to resist a poison (e.g., a pesticide) that normally kills the species. These immunized specimens will survive a fresh application of the poison. They have the enormous biological advantage, furthermore, that as regards propagation in their own biological field they have no competitors. They will therefore, multiply rapidly and a strain will be formed that can no longer be controlled by means of the original pesticide.

The resistance buildup can thus usually be regarded as unavoidable, as it depends on generally valid biological principles. The stronger and more frequent the application of the poison, the faster the resistance develops to the poison. Following the bulk application of chemical pesticides after the Second World War, the number of pest species with powers of resistance increased dramatically. Most of the 600 and more species of pests known today are multiresistant (immune to a variety of pesticides). The increase in the powers of resistance means that ever higher concentrations of poison must be applied and that more and more poisons must be developed.

Another serious ecological consequence of the application of pesticides is the increase in from pressure parasites. On each form of animal life several limiting factors are imposed by nature in the form of disease, natural enemies (insects and animals beneficial to man in destroying pests) and inert organisms. By the application of pesticides these limiting factors are modified or destroyed, so that the road is left open to a mass increase in species of pests. Various factors also result in the insects and animals that help to eliminate the pests being more seriously affected by the pesticides than the pests themselves.

The natural enemies of plant lice such as ladybugs, lacewings and syrphus flies—which in one year may have no more than a few hundred young, whereas under favorable conditions plant lice can multiply several thousands of times in a couple of weeks—are so severely affected by pesticides that their normal low propagation rate is even further reduced. In addition, because of their predatory mobile habits, the insects given to exterminating vermin are far more likely to come into contact with spray poison, even if they were not originally directly sprayed. Many pests, on the other hand, because of their static existence, are often not touched by the pesticide (as they cling to the underside of a leaf, for instance) and survive unscathed.

For these reasons a single application of pesticide may cause disturbance or destruction of the natural controlling factors for parasites. Unnoticed by most people, the numbers of many small and medium-sized creatures such as bumblebees, butterflies beetles and lizards are reduced by the insidious operation of poisons in the environment.

The density of a population (the total number of individuals of one species, race, etc., in a demarcated area) depends on four opposing processes: birthrate, death rate, immigration and emigration. For all forms of animal and plant life, the number of offspring exceeds the number of individuals capable of propagating. This stems from the fact that a number of the individuals die prematurely from disease or attack. This is particularly true of insects. If the proliferation of insects were not reduced by outside factor, there would soon be overpopulation of insects and consequent destruction of the fundamentals of life for the individual.

As such a development could not be of advantage to any species, a number of limiting factors stand in the way of such overproduction. An important limiting factor is the quantity of nutrients available in proportion to the density of population. If the density of population is too high, competitors will contend for the elements of life essential to survival, such as nutrients, breeding grounds and mating partners. The competitive struggle between members of a species is particularly severe, because these all have the same requirements. But competitive struggles also arise between members of different species. A further important limiting factor is the natural enemies (viruses, predators and parasites) of a species.

A great influence on population density is also exerted by external physical factors such as temperature, air humidity, light intensity and strength of winds. Temperature, for instance, can affect the number and development of eggs, but indirectly it can also have an effect on parasites.

In relation to the efficiency of the individual environmental factors, for each form of animal and plant life there is a specific optimum. Thus an apple tree grows best and bears most fruit when the ideal conditions for its species or kind as regards temperature, air humidity and sunshine are present. The same applies to the parasites they prey on the apple tree. A precise knowledge of the individual factors that play a role in population dynamics is essential for the effective biological destruction of insect pests. Especially, if one were to know the curves for the respective ecological optimum of the various useful plants and parasites, which unfortunately is the case today for only particular species. One would then be able to handle the destruction of insect pests more effectively by a favorable choice of location.

Cultural methods can be adopted or revised to exercise an influence, in the landscape and environment, on the population density of parasites in agriculture and forestry. The principle underlying such measures is to render the living conditions of the harmful organisms less favorable, with a view to restricting their propagation and so keeping their population density below the danger threshold. In the long run these preventive measures, by means of which a solitary intervention in the landscape can produce long-term results, may provide the most elegent and at the same time a considerable labor- and energy-saving solution. Their application, however, presupposes a precise knowledge of the ecology of the useful plants concerned and of the harmful organisms affecting them.

The viruses of yellow fever and malaria, for example, are transmitted by mosquitoes. These insects can propagate on a large scale only when they possess sufficient marshland in which the larvae can germinate. By draining their breeding grounds in many countries, yellow fever and malaria outbreaks have thus been reduced drastically.

Many insect pests, especially smaller ones, avoid the wind, as they are easily carried away by it. By planting carrots and cabbages in fields exposed to the wind, it has been possible to reduce the infestation of these cultivated plants by carrot flies and cabbage flies considerably. Especially vulnerable to insect pests are monocultures of a particular species of plant, in which the insects can propagate and multiply unhindered. On the other hand, mixed cultures, in which two more kinds of plants are grown together, offer reasonable possibilities for preventing the spread of insect pests from a fallen plant to a neighbouring one, as the distance between the individual plants of the same kind is increased. An additional safeguard is to place two plants in a mixed culture which protect one another against insect pests.

The planting of carrots and onions together in a mixed culture would thus provide effective protection against the carrot fly and the onion fly, since the onion fly avoids the essential oils of the carrot and the carrot fly avoids the order of the onion. Another very effective method of protecting plants is the cultivation and use of resistant kinds of culture plants. It was thus possible to arrest the severe damage to vineyards in Europe caused by the incursion of the vine louse (Phylloxera) in the second half of the nineteenth century by grafting the European vine onto American stock, which was not vulnerable to the vine louse.

Today there are numerous plants that are not susceptible to the damage from insect pests, such as potatoes that are resistant to viral diseases, and cereal crops that are invulnerable to rust fungi. Nevertheless, efforts in this area in future must be intensified considerably. Another measure for the cultural destruction of insect pests is the planting of shrubs and hedges, which provide birds that prey on insects with cover and a breeding ground. Generally speaking, living communities and landscapes are the more stable against mass propagation of insect pests the more diversified and variegated they are.

The general procedure for cultural defense against insect pests consists, therefore, in increasing the diversity of the landscape and thereby improving its regulation capacity.

An animal is described as beneficial when it serves as the opponent of harmful insect life. The terms *beneficial* and *harmful* are relative in this context, as they are applied by man according to his concept of usefulness. Creatures beneficial to man are classified as *predators*, whose prey is insect pests; *parasites*, which live on insect pests, and *morbific agents* (carriers of a disease), which communicate diseases to insect pests.

Typical predators among beneficial animal and insects are lizards, falcons, bats, wild and domestic cats, various insects such as ground beetles, ladybugs, assassin bugs and their larvae, and the larvae of syrphus flies and of certain gall gnats. The parasites include the tachinds and ichneumons. The fully grown female of the plant-louse ichneumon will thus lay an egg in th full-fledged plant louse. The larva produced from the egg will feed for a couple of days on the inside of the plant louse. It will then pupate in the plant louse and after a short time an inchneumon will slip from the empty shell of the plant louse and, after mating, will soon lay more eggs in other plant lice. Although only one plant louse is killed each time by the ichneumon larva, because of the high propagation rate a sizable plant louse population can be exterminated in a relatively short time.

In the group of morbific (pathogenic) agents are included viruses and microorganisms such as fungi, bacteria and protozoa which can communicate to the insect pests on which they prey an infectious disease that usually proves fatal. Once the disease of the particular organisms are identified, the pathogenic agent can be isolated, cultivated intensively and applied to the biological destruction of insect pests.

In connection with biological destruction of pests by animals and insects, a number of important factors have to be considered. In the first place, a particular animal species is regarded as a serious parasite only when the depredations for which it is responsible exceed a certain economic threshold. This occurs when measures taken to reduce mass propagation of the parasite are dropped. In normal conditions of ecolgical equilibrium, each species of organism is subject to certain limiting factors that are hardly discernible to the inexperienced observer, in the form in particular of the organism's natural enemies. This becomes increasingly obvious when the natural enemies of the parasite are unintentionally so incapacitated by spraying with toxic pesticides that they can no longer perform their role as limiting factors in the propagation of parasitc life.

In certain circumstances one single spraying may be enough to upset the ecological equilibrium of a life community so severely that a proliferation of parasites will result. Everything possible should therefore be done to preserve the ecological equilibrium of nature or, insofar as it have been disrupted by agriculture, forestry and horticulture, to restore it to some extent.

An important ecological contribution can be made by the syrphus fly, for example. Its larvae suck out the insides of plant lice and so keep their population density down. The mature insect itself bears some resemblance to the wasp, in that its yellow, white or orange abdomen has black or dark brown stripes, according to the species to which it belongs. These extremely adopt flying creatures can switch from zigzag dashes at lightning speed to remaining suspended, with wings still buzzing, at some point in the air. In contrast to their larvae, they are attracted to flowering plants and feed on nectar. Thus if flowering plants are available in sufficient quantities, enough syrphus fly larvae should be present in a given area for the biological reduction of plant lice. In areas of intensive fruit and vegetable cultivation, in which every weed is treated with herbicides, the flowering plants are not present. It is not surprising, therefore, that no beneficial syrphus fly larvae are to be found here.

And strange though this may seem, the presence of a certain number of insect pests during the entire vegetation period may also prove beneficial, for only in this way can the presence of their predators be assured. The best guarantee that insect pests are available in small numbers (below the economic damage threshold) is ecological versatility with as many varieties of plants as possible and numerous ecological niches. Provided there are sufficient weeds available for the numerous insect pests (who will not yet be endangering the useful plants), the survival of the beneficial insects is assured. As beneficial insects are very sensitive to toxic chemical spraying, they are eliminated in most cases more rapidly and in greater numbers than the destructive pests for which it is intended. In addition, the pest insects recover more rapidly, as they usually have a shorter generation gap than their predators and are present in much greater profusion.

Creatures that can play a useful part in the biological elimination of parasites include ladybugs with their larvae, syrphus fly larvae, ichneumon flies, and assassin bugs; against fruit-tree parasites (especially caterpillars) many birds, such as the titmouse; earwings are particularly partial to palt lice and the coddling moth; enemies of the mouse include the falcons and the weasel; and the widest varieties of ichneumons live in particular cases on a very specific type of insect pest. The viruses to which individual pests are prone have been investigated to only a very limited extent.

The great advantage of the biological destruction of insect pests, as opposed to their destruction by chemical means, lies in the fact that it does not impair the quality of foodstuffs. Viruses had parasites tend to attach themselves to a particular host, and so remain completely neutral with regard to other animals and to human beings. Another advantage of biological destruction of pests consists in the cheapness and simplicity of its methods. No complicated machinery is required for applying it and no great labour costs are incurred in frequent spraying. The biological destruction of pests leaves nature to do its work and makes full use of natural principles.

Many animal species secrete particular stimulating substances, known as pheromones, which influence relations between individual members. They are most strongly developed in gregarious species such as ants, bees, mice, rats. But they also occur in nongregarious groups in the form of sexual lures which affect only the mating partner. Thorough investigations have been made recently into pheromones for insects. These substances are effective for the most part in extremely low concentrations; the male of the American cockroach, for instance, reacts to a mere 30 molecules of the sexual lure emitted by the mating partner. Such substances can be perceived over areas many kilometers in extent. It has now been possible to isolate the sexual pheromones of the following pests among others: coddling moths. Asiatic cotton worms, sugarcane bugs, night moths, various bark beetles and various kinds of moth that imperil the corn crop.

In principle there are two possibilities for controlling damage by pheromones:

1. The lure substance, extracted from the animal or produced synthetically, is inserted in traps or snares, into which the male of the species concerned is thus enticed. One example of this is the bark beetle, the pheromones of which can be reproduced

synthetically. When this lure substance, which affects both sexes, is inserted in selected tree traps, the bark beetles in the vicinity are attracted. By felling these lure trees and removing the bark, the pupa of the beetle can be readily destroyed. The use of sexual pheromones for pest control by this method is likely to succeed, however, only when the population density of the pest in the locality concerned is low, so that the lure substance in the traps will not be masked by the lure substance of the particular insect.

2. By large-scale distribution of a lure substance during the nuptial flight of butterflies and moths, the males of the species can be so confused that they can no longer locate the female with its similar emission of pheromone. This process was put to the test successfully for the first time in the United States in connection with control of the vegetable owl (*Mamestra oleracea*) caterpillars. In this case a concentration of about 10^{-10} grams of pheromone per gram of air was used. In order to maintain this concentration, about 1.5 grams of substance, were needed per hectare per night.

In contrast to the lure substances, certain odiferous agents given off by many plants have a repellent effect on various insects. Such repellents can be employed for plant protection in one of two ways: (1) The repellents from particular resistant plant forms can be isolated, or produced synthetically, and then sprayed over the field of cultivated plants in need of protection. From resistant species of potatoes, for instance, glucosides such as solanine and tomatine can be isolated, which act as deterrents to potato beetles. (2) Very much simpler is the method of siting plants that emit repellents in a mixed culture with selected useful plants, so that attacks by pests on the useful plants are avoided. If tomatoes and cabbages are grown in this way in mixed cultures, the repellents emitted by the tomatoes will prevent attacks on the cabbage plants by caterpillars of the cabbage butterfly.

Ecological weed Control

There are various methods for restricting the growth of weeds. Chemical weed-killers (herbicides) are used for the most part, especially in agriculture. They are sprayed on the weeds, which wither away under their effects. The herbicides can also have unfortunate incidental effects on other plants, however, and so on the quality of food crops. For this reason a switch to ecological methods of weed control is to be recommended. Basically, this can be done in three ways: by mechanical means, by the employment of animals that devour weeds.

1. By working the soil (clearing it of weeds, plowing, etc.), the weeds can be exterminated or destroyed by mechanical means. This traditional method is very expensive labourious, however.
2. Great success has been achieved by the employment of animals that consume weeds as fodder. Some imported weeds have been treated in this way. One example among many is the reduction of the prickly-pear cactus (Opuntia) in parts of Australia. About the year 1840 several Opuntia species were imported from Central America into the Australian states of Queensland and New South Wales, where they grew unexpectedly and by 1925, covered an area of some 24 million hectares. From 1913, attempts were made to check the spread of these cacti. Of some 160 animal species from North and South America known to prey on the prickly pear, 48 species were examined in a quarantine station for possibilities of damage to the ecological equilibrium of their new habitat. Of the 23 species ultimately

released, 13 species (12 insect species and 1 mite) were able to propagate. Most successful was an Argentine small butterfly, the caterpillars of which ate seams out of the cacti, while putrefactive bacteria resulted in the death of the cacti. By 1936, a stretch of land in Queensland that had previously been overgrown by a dense cactusthicket was practically cleared of the weeds, and in New South Wales up to 10% more land was available for cultivation.

3. Eradication of weeds by other plants is based on the assumption that the plants that supersede are not in the nature of weeds themselves but have the effect, as far as possible, of improving the soil conditions.As the term weed is purely relative, many plants can have a harmful, neutral or beneficial effect on the cultivated plants and the soil according to their nature and conditions. For the most part a plant has a weed effect if it has a thick root structure which restricts the root growth of useful plants and deprives them of nutrients and trace elements. If a thick-rooted plant is replaced by one with light roots, which allow developing plants to germinate, and if by symbiosis with root bacteria combining with atmospheric nitrogen (as in the case of papilionaceous, or leguminous, flowers) it contributes to improving the soil by enriching it with nitrogen compounds, in most cases the weed problem will be solved. Covering the ground with an intermediate fruit growth of this order will also help to prevent drying out of the soil. The growth of microorganisms and the living conditions of earthworms that help to break up the soil are also promoted in this way. For these reasons the suppression of weeds by introducing other plants to the area is certainly the most presentable and ecologically most satisfactory method of weed control.

The environmental problems associated with the extensive use of slowly degrading pesticides have been appreciated for many years. Large quantities of these compounds are being manufactured and deliberately distributed in the environment to control plant and insect pests. The environmental stability of many of these compound has been highly appreciable. However, the toxicity and environmental problems associated with the commercial use of other haloorganics that get accidentally released into the environment has only recently been appreciated. For example, polychlorinated biphenyls (PCBs) have been extremely stable industrial compounds with an environmental half-life of about 15 years. Another example has been vinyl chloride (chloroethene), which has been probably almost as stable as the PCBs get lost in to the environment each year in the process of manufacturing of polyvinyl chloride plastic.

As vinyl chloride is a gas at room temperature, this compound probably occurs mainly as an atmospheric containment. Vinyl chloride was used as an aerosol propellant but this use was banned because it was found that the vinyl chloride monomer was responsible for a rate type of liver cancer and may be responsible for birth defects. There is suspicion that other vinyl chloride derivatives such as 1, 1-dichloroethylene and trichloroethylene, are also carcinogens. 1, 1-dichloroethylene finds use in the manufacture of the plastic Saran Wrap while trichloroethylene finds use extensively for the degreasing of metal parts in metal fabricating plants. No estimates have been made on the release of trichloroethylene in the environment.

Yet another example of a hazardous halocarbon has been 1, 2-dibromo-3 chloropropane. This has caused sterility in the males exposed to this chemical in the course of its manufacture. Therefore, its manufacture has been banned. A potential environmental problem of a different kind has been arisen from the extensive use of fluorochlorocarbons (Freons) as propellants in aerosol cans and as the refrigerants in refrigeration systems. Because of the volatility of these fluorocarbons, they are present almost exclusively in the atmosphere.

Freons and carbon tetrachloride are not susceptible to environmental degradation until they reach the stratosphere where they are photodissociated by ultra-violet light. This process is responsible for the partial destruction of the ozone layer. Even a partial loss of the ozone layer could result in a dangerous increase in the amount of ultravoilet light reaching the surface of the earth. A different source of environmental chloroorganic compounds is the chlorination of drinking water. Some of the organic compounds present in water can get chlorinated by this procedure. It is well established that chloroform, bromo-dichloromethane, dibromochlo-romethane, and bromoform are produced in the process of chlorination if appropriate materials are present.

In addition both carbon tetrachloride and 1, 2-dichloroethane have been detected in the drinking water. Although it is believed that both chloroform and carbon tetrachloride are carcinogens, the amounts present in the drinking water (up to 311 ppb for chloroform) are probably not sufficient for including tumor formation. While chlorinated organic materials are among the most widely used pesticides, their overall environmental impact coupled with the development of insect resistance to their effects, give rise to increasing use of other classes of compounds for pesticidal purposes. Some aspects of the chemistry of the most important and typical of these other classes will be described in this chapter.

Organochlorine derivatives may be prepared industrially by the direct chlorination of hydrocarbons.

$$RH+Cl_2 \rightarrow RCl+HCl \quad ...(1)$$

Chlorination finds use in the preparation of orgaanochlorine compounds such as 1, 3-dichloro-1-propene, which are effective in killing nematodes (soil worms). The overall reaction is

$$CH_2 = CHC_3+2Cl_2 \rightarrow ClCH{=}CHCH_2Cl{=}2HCl \quad ...(2)$$

Aromatic compounds generally have been more difficult to chlorinate than aliphatic compounds. Polychlorinated biphenyls may be prepared from biphenyl by direct chlorination using ferric chloride as a catalyst.

Polychlorinated biphenyls may be produced by the chlorination of wastes in sewage disposal plants that had an appreciable input of biphenyl from a textile mill. This indicates that the use of chlorine in waste treatment may be dangerous because environmentally stable organochlorine compounds may get formed.

Polychlorinated Biphenyls

Introduction Polychlorinate biphenyls have been available commercially for over 40 years. The synthesis from chlorine and biphenyl yields a mixture of derivatives with the extent of chlorination being dependent on the chlorine-biphenyl ratio.

PCBs are resistant to acid, base, heat and oxygen. This extreme stability makes them especially useful as a dielectric material in capacitors and transformers. They have also been used as plasticizers and solvents in plastics and printing inks. Closely related compounds, polybrominated biphenyls, are used as flame retardants.

Sources of PCBs in the Environment. Although PCBs may be formed in some instances in sewage treatment plants and by the photolyses of DDT derivatives, undoubtedly industrially produced PCBs are the main environmental source. It is estimated that 4000 tons per year enter the environment from the dumping and leaking of lubricants heat transfer fluids, and hydraulic fluids into rivers and streams. Another 1000-2000 tons per year were discharge into the atmosphere by the combustion of plastics containing PCBs as plasticilizers. As PCBs are resistant to combustion, they were merely volatized during the incineration.

Environmental Degradation. The environmental breakdown of PCBs is exceedingly slow with a half-life estimated to be 10-15 years. The mechanism for this breakdown is not known. Recently it has been reported that lightly chlorinated PCBs are hydroxylated by rats and pigeons but not by brook trout, as indicated in reaction (4) and (5). The hydroxylation reaction is reminiscent of the hydroxylations catalyzed by the aryl oxidase enzyme cytochrome P-450. Since similar oxidations are effected by microorganisms, it is conceivable that lightly chlorinated PCBs are also degraded in this way environmentally, although the highly chlorinated ones have been certainly much more resistant.

Toxicity. PCBs do not exhibit significant immediate (acute) toxicity and have been considered to be nontoxic. However, toxic effects were amply demonstrated in 1968 when more than 1000 persons in Japan ate rice oil contaminated with PCBs that had leaked into the oil from a heat exchanger. Those persons who ate 0.5 gm or more (average consumption was 2 gm) developed darkened skin, eye damage, and severe acne. It is not sure if the subsequent deaths of some of the patients were due to the PCB poisoning. Recovery was slow with symptoms still present even after ten years. Several infants were born with the same symptoms, demonstrating the PCBs can readily cross the plocental barrier. PCBs have been found to be toxic to mink and some species of shellfish, shrimp, and fish. The chronic (long term) toxicity of PCBs and other chloroorganics has been described elsewhere in the chapter.

DDT

Synthesis. DDT (1, 1, 1-trichloro-2, 2-bis (p-chlorophenyl) ethane, also called dichlorodiphenyltrichloromethane, hence the name DDT], is obtained by the reaction of chloral with chlorobenzene. The p, p^{-1}-isomer shown is not the only reaction product. Appreciable amounts of o, p'-and o, o'-DDT are also obtained. This synthetic approach has been applied for the preparation of a great variety of DDT analogs. One important example, methoxychlor, is currently being used in place of DDT in many applications because it is biodegradable. However, it is less effective as an insecticide and about three times as costly to prepare because anisole (methoxybenzene) is a more expensive starting material than chlorobenzene.

Environmental Degradation. DDT undergoes a relatively rapid elimination of HCL to yield DDE [1, 1-dichloro-2, 2-bis (p-chlorophenyl) ethylene] when heated in water. However, the subsequent hydrolysis of DDE is extremely slow because there are only unreactive vinyl and aryl chlorides in DDE. As a consequence, DDE is the principal DDT degradation product found in the environment. Methoxychlor and other DDT analogs that do not have the p, p′-cloro group have been much less persistent in the environment. This is due to their metabolism by soil microorganisms to phenols that are readily degraded further to acetate.

The enzymes involved in these oxidations have been probably of the cytochroma P-450 type mentioned previously. Similar enzymes are present in insects. The lower toxicity of methoxychlor as compared to DDT may reflect the effective oxidative detoxification of methoxychlor by some insects.

Mechanism of Action of DDT and DDT Analogs. Insects sprayed with DDT exhibit hyperactivity and convulsions consistent with the interaction of the DDT with the nervous system. Many theories have been postulated for the toxic effect of DDT and the exact mechanism is not known. A current theory that appears plausible and has some experimental basis is that the DDT molecules are of the correct size to get trapped in the pores of the nerve membranes. This distorts the membrane and sodium ions leak through and depolarize the nerve cell so that it can no longer transmit impules. This theory states that the toxicity of DDT is not attributed to its chemical reactivity but rather to its size and geometry that allows for the blockage of the pores of the nerve membranes. This theory has been supported by the observation that a variety of quite different compounds that are stereochemically similar to DDT exhibit DDT exhibit DDT-like activity.

The special fit hypothesis has been further supported by the observation that the biological acativity of methoxychlor analogs gets decreased rapidly when R in the formula below contain five carbon atoms or more. Presumably the longerchain methoxychlor analogs have not been able to fit in the nerve pores.

Insects are especially susceptible to DDT because it is readily absorbed through the insect cuticle. DDT is not appreciably absorbed through the protein skin of mammals. If the polarity of the DDT analog is increased by introducing -NO_2, -CO_2H, - CO_2CH_3, and - OH substituents into the aromatic ring, the toxicity is lost. This loss is probably due in part to decreased absorption through the cuticle and in part to decreased adsorption on the nonpolar nerve membrane.

Insect Resistance to DDT. When DDT came into widespread use after World War II, it appeared to be the answer for the control of all insects. However, as early as 1948 there were reports that it was no longer as effective as it had previously been. It was subsequently found that DDT-resistant flies and mosquitoes were still susceptible to dieldrin and lindane although in a few years, resistance developed for these pesticides as well. It was observed that DDT-resistant flies were "knocked down" by normal doses of DDT, but after some buzzing around on the floor they eventually recovered. This observation suggested that the resistant strains have a mechanism for rapidly detoxifying the DDT. Subsequent investigations revealed that DDT-resistant strains contained an enzyme (DDT dehydrochlorinase) that was not present in those flies that were susceptible to DDT, and that it catalyzed the conversion of DDT to DDE.

Aninteresting result that is consistent with the proposed action of DDT dehydrochlorinase is the observation that a deuterium-substituted DDT derivative shown below is more effective than DDT against resistant strains, yet it exhibits the same level of toxic effect against non-resistant strains as DDT. The enzymic dehydrochlorination of DDT probably procceeds by an E2 mechanism with the C-H (or C-D) and C-Cl bonds broken in the rate-limiting step [reaction (7)]. However, removal of the deuterium by base is slower than proton removal because of the greater strength of C-D bond (1.2 kcal/mole greater) as compared to the C-H bond (a deuterium isotope effect). Since the deuterated analog is converetd to DDE more slowly by DDT dehydrochlorinase, it has a greater time to exert its toxic effect on the resistant strain.

Insect resistance to insecticides is a commonly observed phenomenon. Resistance develops where 100% insect mortality does not occur and where just sublethal doses of the insecticide remain in the vicinity for long periods of time. The surviving insects breed under these conditions and only those progeny that are resistant to the residual insecticide survive. In this way a resistant strain develops that is able to survive in the presence the insecticide. Resistance is not observed as frequently with those insecticides that are destroyed rapidly in the environment. A non-resistant population of insects may build up again when the insecticide is no longer used. This occurs if the non-resistant strain (wild type) adapts more successfully to the insecticide-free environment than the resistant strain. However a population of resistant insects forms very rapidly if the insecticide is reintroduced.

Knowledge of the mechanism of toxic action, the pathways for environmental degradation, and the cause of insect resistance should allow for the synthesis of environmentally degradable DDT analogs that are active against resistant strains. More sophisticate pesticides can be designed once the complexities of the molecular reactions and interactions are understood. However, resistance will always be a problem and it is highly unlikely that insects can be controlled exclusively with synthetic insecticides.

Synthesis. Lindane is prepared by the free radical addition of chlorine atoms to benzene. Of the eight possible isomers, only four are formed in appreciable amounts [reaction (10)]. These isomers differ in the relative orientations of the chloro substituents. Axial (a) groups are perpendicular to the cyclohexane ring and are labeled in the a-isomer in (10). Equatorial groups are in the equatorial plane of the ring as shown in the β-isomer. Only one of these isomers, the y-isomer, exhibits significant insecticidal action. Initially, the total reaction mixture was used as the insecticide. However, that practice has been discontinued because this results in the distribution of large amounts of inactive chlorocarbon compounds in the environment. The use of lindane is quite restricted in many countries. It tends to accumulate in the fatty tissues of mammals, thus it is no longer used in animal husbandary. It is used to control limited insect infestations such as borers, beetles, and hornets and it has been used in flea collars.

Polychlorinated Cyclopentadience Derivatives

Synthesis. A series of bicyclic insecticides, chlordane, heptachlor, aldrin, and dieldrin, can be synthesized by the Diels-Alder addition of hexachlorocyclopentadiene to olefins. The preparation of these compounds is shown in reactions (12 to 14). Obviously it is possible to prepare a whole series of potential insecticides by this route by simply varying the diene and olefin.

The endo-adduct (see structure below) is major product resulting from the Diels-Alder addition of a diene and an olefin.

Environment Degradation. The cyclopentadiene insecticide are very resistant to environmental forces. One might expect that the tetiary, allylic chloro groups would be especially susceptible to SN 1 hydrolsis or E1 elimination. However, the rigid geometry of the bicyclic ring system prevents carbonium ion formation, as shown in reaction 15. A carbonium ion is more stable if positive central carbon atom and the three substituents attached to it are in the same plane. It is not possible to obtain a plannar carbonium ion intermediate at the bridgehead carbon atom of these compounds without introducing extraordinary strain in the bicyclic system.

These compounds are susceptible to oxidative attack by soil microorganism, plants, and animals. However, the resulting products, such as the one illustrated in reaction

(16), are often more toxic than the starting pesticide. Photodieldrin (17) is formed by the action of ultraviolet light as well as by the action of oxidase enzymes on dieldrin. The mechanism of action of these bicyclic organoclorins compounds' is similar to that of DDT. However, the effects of these compounds suggest that the site of action is the ganglia of the central nervous system rather than the peripheral nerves that are affected by DDT. The manufacture of aldrin and dieldrin has been banned in many countries because of their potential danger as carcinogens. Preliminary evidence suggests that heptachlor and chloroane are also carcinogens-a not unexpected result in view of their structural similarity to aldrin and dieldrin.

2. 4-Dichlorophenoxyacetic Acid (2, 4-D) and 2, 4, 5-Trichlorophenoxyacetic Acid (2, 4, 5-T)

Intr›duction. 2, 4-D and 2, 4, 5-T have been herbicides that have been especially effective in the control of broad-leafed plants yet they have little or no effect on grasses. Hence they find use to control weeds and other unwanted vegetation.

These compounds mimic the plant growth hormone (auxin) indoleacetic acid, but the large amounts used (compared to the natural auxin) being about abnormal growth of the plant. In particular, little or no root growth, abnormal stem growth, and leaves with little or no chlorophyll are observed.

Synthesis. 2, 4-D and 2, 4,.5-T may be manufactured by the SN_2 displacement of the chloro group of chlorocetate with a phenoxide anion or by the chlorination of phenoxyacetic acid. Numerous closely related 2, 4-D analogs also shows herbicidal activity. The carboxyl can be replaced by the amide, nitrile, or ester groups. In addition, a longer side chain can be used in place of the acetic acid moiety. However, this side chain must have an even number of carbon atoms. to be active. This result has been in consistent with β-oxidation of the side chain in the plant to form the biologically active 2, 4-D.

Environmental Degradation. Pure 2, 4-D and 2, 4, 5-T are subject to rapid environmental degradation. These compounds get readily cleaved by microorganisms to the corresponding phenol which is readily degraded further. Presumably, oxalic acid is the other reaction product. In addition, the photochemical cleavage of the acetic acid side chain and the photochemical hydrolysis of the aryl chloro groups has been demonstrated. These data reveal that the long-term environmental impact of these compounds has been small.

The environmental problem which has been associated with these compounds is due to dioxin impurities produced during their manufacture (25). Dioxins get formed in small amounts during the synthesis of 2, 4-dichlorophenol and 2, 4, 5-trichlorophenol (24) and are carried along with the final product. The dioxins are formed because of the vigorous conditions that are required to hydrolyze the aryl chloro groups.

Related toxic five membered ring derivatives (dibenzofurans) formed in the manufacture of PCBs could be responsible for the toxicity of these compounds. Polybromobiphenyls (PBB) exhibit similar toxic effects to PCBs. This toxicity may occur due in part to trace amounts of brominated dibenzodioxins and dibenzofurans in the PBBs, but this posssibility requires verification. The dioxins produced during the manufacture of 2, 4, 5,-T have been shown to be toxic, teratogenic (cause birth defects) acnegenic in laboratory animals. The acnegenic effect has been observed in workers involved in the manufacture of 2, 4, 5-T. Similar toxic effects were noted with tetrachlorodibedzodioxin. The preliminary results suggest that dioxins may accumulate in the food chain and constitute a health hazard. This possibility is suggested by the observation that there appears to be a greater number of stillbirths, placental tumors, and malformations where the 2, 4, 5-T defoliants were used in Vietnam.

The biochemical cause of the toxicity of dioxins is not known, but two different acnegenic effects have been correlated with the induction of two different enzymes. Higher levels of cytochrome p 450 are induced by dioxins and structurally related tetrachlroazo benzene derivatives. A direct correlation between the ability to produce chloracne and the affinity for the binding sites specific for p-450 induction was observed. Acne associated with enhanced levels of porphyrins is also caused by dioxins because of increased levels of 8-aminolevulinic acid synthetase, an enzyme responsible for one of the steps in porphyrin biosynthesis.

Long-Term Effects of Organochlorine Compounds

The chronic (long-term) toxicity of chlorinated hydrocarbons has been the main problem arising from their use. This toxic effect was first discovered when it was observed that the populations of eagles, hawks falcons, policans, and other bird at the ends of a food chain were decreasing. Closer examination revealved that the birds were mating later in the season and were producing eggs with much thinner shells than normal. Analysis of the birds and their eggs revealed that they contained large amounts of organochlorine compounds. Laboratory studies confirmed that when birds were fed DDT and PCBs, they produced eggs with thin shells.

The cause of the delayed mating has been traced to the enhanced levels of the cytochrome P-450 oxidase enzymes in the livers of those birds containing the organochlorine residues. Enhanced levels of oxidase enzymes are known to be induced by barbiturates and polycyclic aromatic compounds. It was found that DDT, DDE, dieldrin, and PCBs also cause such an enhancement.

The enhancement of the oxidase enzymes affects mating behaviour because these enzymes catalyze the oxidation of steroid hormones. Specifically it was found that an increase in the oxidase enzymes resulted in a decrease in the levels of estradiol in the birds. It is known that the birds will mate only if a certain levels of estradiol is present. If breeding gets delayed, then the offspring hatch at a time when there is less food available for their growth. This is an especially important factor with large birds that require a full season for the young to develop. The production of egg shells has been also influenced by estradiol. The shell of an egg is only formed in the last day before laying. About 60% of the calcium needed to form the egg is obtained from the birds food intake and the remainder-comes from calcium stored in the bone marrow.

As the level of calcium deposited in the bone is regulated by levels of estradiol in the blood, a low level of estradiol results in a low level of stored calcium. The absence of stored calcium could be a significant factor in egg survival since a 20% decrease in shell thickness results in extensive egg breakage. A 20% decrease takes place with as little as 25 ppm of chlororganics in the egg.

Finally, it is observed that some pesticides are able to inhibit the formation of eggshells in the presence of an adequate supply of calcium. Presumably these pesticides interfere with the enzyme carbonic anhydrase that is responsible for the conversion of carbon dioxide to carbonate. The latter is required to combine with calcium to form the calcium carbonate of the shell. So far it has been established that DDE but not dieldrin interfere with the formation of the shell in this way. The chronic toxicity of chloroorganics has not been limited to birds. Mink are highly susceptible to PCBs with level of 5 parts per billion (ppb) sufficient to halt their reproduction. This is an economic problem as mink ranchers have been using Great Lakes coho salmon for mink feed. However, this can no longer be used since the salmon contains 5 ppb PCBs. At present, there are no reports of chronic toxicity of PCBs and chlorinated insecticides in man, but there are some indications that it may exist.

The first is the observation that pesticides induce high levels of liver enzymes in a wide array of vertebrates including the monkey. It seems very likely. that such induction will be observed in man as well. Secondly, it has been observed that a dose of 46 mg/kg of DDT can produce a fourfold increase in tumors in animals. These data suggest a correlation between the ingestion of DDT and cancer. In addition, there is a growing list of chlorinated organic compounds that are known to produce tumors. Obviously, man is in as vulnerable a position as the predatory birds in the food chain so that it may be essential for his survival that he reduce the level of chlorinated hydrocarbons in the environment.

Chlorinated hydrocarbons are ubiquitous in the environment. Residues have been found in locations and in species where chloroorganics have never been used; for example, they have been found in the polar ice pack, in animlas in arctic regions, and in the air over the centre of the ocean. The chlorinated hydrocarbons must be carried through the atmosphere to achieve such wide distribution. The detection of chlorinated hydrocarbons in rainwater has been consistent with this observation. Furthermore, DDT is sufficiently volatile that all that has been manufactured to date could be volatilized and still not saturate the atmosphere. The global circulation of chlorinated hydrocarbons demonstrates that all nations have a stake in the reduction in the manufacture of the international control of chloroorganics.

Application as Pesticides. These organophosphorus compounds exhibit high insecticidal action against a wide variety of species. This is not really an asset because these compounds are highly toxic to vertebrates as well as to insects and, as a consequence, are much more dangerous to the workers using them than are chloroorganics. Demeton is unique in that it shows systemic action. That is, it is absorbed by the plant and its toxic effect is retained in the plant for 1-1.5 months. Obviously, this insecticide is mainly useful for ornamental plants and shrubs that are not consumed as animal or human food-Malathion can be used safely by home gardeners because it is readily detoxified by vertebrates.

The ester groups are readily detoxified by vertebrates. The ester groups are readily hydrolyzed by the esterase enzymes present in mammals but absent in insects. The lethal dose for killing 50% of the mammals ingesting it (LD_{50}) is 500-1500 mg/kg of body weight for malathion as compared to an LD_{50} of 6-12 mg/kg for parathion and 25-50 mg/kg for methyl parathion.

The toxic effect of the organophosphorus insecticides is due to their interference in the transfer of nerve impulses from one nerve cell to the next. When a nerve impulse reaches the end of a nerve cell it triggers the release of a minute amount of the compound acetylcholine. The acetylcholine activates a receptor on an adjacent nerve cell causing it to carry the impulse to the next nerve cell. The acetylcholine is then hydrolyzed to choline and acetic acid by the enzyme cholinesterase as in reaction (32). Other enzymes then reconstitute the choline and acetic acid to acetylcholine on the nerve endings. The organophosphorous pesticides bind chemically to the cholinesterase so that it can no longer catalyze the hydrolysis of acetylcholine. The resulting excess of acetylcholine hyperstimulates nerves and produces convulsions, irregular heartbeat, and choking in vertebrates.

Environmental Degradation. The organophosphorus insecticide undergo a very rapid hydrolysis in the environment. This is a mixed blessing. There is no build up of residues; however, frequent application of the pesticide is required. Some typical hydrolytic reactions include reactions (33) to (35). The nitro group of parathion is reduced by soil microorganisms to give the non-toxic aminoparathion, which is stable and remains bound to the soil. It is not known if this "inactive" form of parathion constitutes an environmental problem.

A problem associated with these organophosphorus insecticides is their environmental conversion to more toxic substances. For example, demeton-O, the by-product formed in the synthesis of demeton-S [reaction (30)] has an LD_{50} of 2 mg/kg for vertebrates as compared to an LD_{50} of 100 mg/kg for demeton-S. The demeton rearrangement takes place readily in plant tissues and may explain the long term systemic action of demeton. If the rearranged product is really the toxic agent, then trace amounts would still be effective. Parathion readily gets oxidized by atmospheric oxygen or enzymatically to a derivative that is four times as toxic as parathion itself. Since parathion exhibits on anticholinesterase activity itself, its insecticidal action may be ascribed to its enzymatic conversion to the oxygen analog in the insect.

Carbaryl. The carbamate insecticide carbaryl has been used extensively as a replacement for DDT to control the gypsy moth as well as other insects. Its toxicity to insects is due to its anticholinesterase action. It is not very toxic to mammals (LD_{50} for rats is 0.5 gm/kg) presumably because it is readily oxidized and excreted, Carbaryl is not persistent in the environment because it is rapidly destroyed by number of pathways and as a consequence it must be applied frequently for insect control. Some of the key reactions of this material have been given in reactions (37) to 39).

Captan. It finds use as a broad-spectrum protective fungicide for the control of diseases of agricultural crops. It is essentially non-toxic with an LD_{50} for rats of 9 gm/kg. Captan undergoes ready hydrolysis by water [reaction (40)] so it does not persist in the environment. The fungicidal action may be due to alkylation of the various sulphydryl groups in the fungus cell by the reactive trichloromethylthio group.

It is a herbicide which finds use to control perennial and annual weeds that are difficult to control with other compounds. It is fairly long-lived with a half-life in soil of 18 months. It has been shown to get destroyed photo chemically in laboratory studies. The decarboxylation product of picrolam has been isolated (41) along with two monodehalogenated products of unknown structure. Picrolam is having a very low toxicity with an LD_{50} of 2.8 gm/kg in a variety of experimental animals.

Atrazine and Simazine. These are derivatives of symmetrical triazine that find use for the control of weeds in corn. Atrazine and simazine are relatively nontoxic compounds with and LD_{50} for rats of 3 gm/kg or greater. Microorganisms are responsible for the environmental degradation of these compounds, but this is a slow process since their half-life in soil samples is 10-12 months. The first step involves cleavage of the N-alkyl grouping [reaction (42)]. The hydrolytic cleavage of the

C-Cl bond to form the C-OH group has been another decomposition pathway. Recent studies have revealed that atrazine may enhance or suppress the toxicity of DDT and parathion depending on the soil type, concentration of pesticides and other environmental factors. The reason for this effect is not clear. It is often observed that the biological effect of a mixture of pesticides is not the sum of the effects of the individual components of the mixture.

Diquat and Paraquat. The bipyridylium herbicides dequat and paraquat are used for the nonselective eradication of plants prior to the planting of a crop and for the control of aquatic plant. They are able to kill the green leaves on which they are applied but cannot penetrate mature bark and so they may be used to control weeds in orchards. They work most rapidly in the presence of strong sunlight. The compounds are relatively toxic to mammals with an LD_{50} of 30-300 mg/kg for oral dose. However, the quaternary salts are not absorbed through the skin so they are not hazardous to man.

These compounds serve as herbicides because they are capable of being reduced in plants to free radicals. The energy for this reduction comes from photosynthesis. The free radicals get reoxidized readily back to the original quaternary ions generating hydrogen peroxide or other radicals that destroy the plant cell.

9 ENVIRONMENTAL CONTROL

Land is the basic resource for providing the needs of the people. Land degradation is an important environmental problem. It is estimated that nearly 100 million hectares of land, almost one-third of the total area, have been affected by land degradation caused by soil erosion, salinity, alkalinity, wind erosion etc. Out of the 300 million hectares of land available in the country only about 150 million hectares is cropped. The productivity of the land has to increase from the present 150 MT to 275 MT in order to feed the population by the year 2000.

Soil erosion is a matter of serious concern to India. Deforestation and cultivation of marginal lands have, it is estimated, led to a loss of 6000 million tonnes of soil annually resulting in loss of productivity. The livestock population of India has increased from about 280 million in 1951 to about 375 million.

About 13 million hectares of land is classified as pastures but much of this has been diverted to agriculture by the poor and most of the rest is degraded. Animals have to scrounge for whatever they can get on the fallow lands and on forest lands. Overgrazing has led to further land degradation.

Deforestation

The forests of India occupy an area of about 75 million hectares, i.e. 22 per cent of the land area. These forests supply the demands of people for timber, fuelwood and minor forest products. However, with the increase in human and cattle population the biotic pressures have become intense.

In addition, industrialisation has brought about increase in demand for wood. In the early years of independence the degraded forest land was diverted for agricultural purposes. In addition, development projects such as hydro-electric projects and industries claimed their share of forest land. A combined result of these causes has reduced the forest cover to about 19 per cent of the area between 1972 and 1982.

The average annual water resource of India is estimated to about 400 million hectare metres (MHM). Out of this, however, about 300 MHM is received by rainfall during the four months of monsoon. The vegetation cover which existed in earlier times used to hold back the monsoon waters and release them steadily after augmenting the ground water. With deforestation, this cushion is gradually disappearing and the water availability is becoming uneven. A high rainfall would result in a flood while a deviation below the normal would create a drought. Floods carry the soil with them leading to silting of rivers and reservoirs.

This alternating cycle of floods and droughts has been steadily increasing. The annual expenditure on meeting the floods and droughts has reached a level of Rs. 1500 crores. Industrialisation has posed a threat to water quality through effluents discharged from industries. Untreated human wastes from towns and cities reach the water courses . These discharges affect the quality of surface water and ground water.

The problems of air pollution are beginning to be felt in India with the accelerated industrial tempo. A survey of the cities has revealed problems of excessive sulphur dioxide in some locations. Automobile pollution is becoming a problem in metropolitan cities, particularly in Delhi and Bombay.

India is very rich in biological diversity with about 45,000 species of plants and 75,000 animal species. These genetic resources are the most precious assets which are now threatened by human encroachment. Protection of this natural heritage is an environmental challenge facing the country. Energy is critical to all development activities covering the household, agriculture, transport and industrial sectors. The rate of commercial energy consumption has more than doubled during the last 40 years, especially in industry and transport sectors.

However, most of the people of India still depend on biomass-based energy such as fuelwood and agricultural wastes. The crisis due to deforestation and indiscriminate cutting down of trees has affected this source of cheap energy.

India's growing population and rapid urbanisation have resulted in an enormous burden on human settlements. By the year 2000, the urban population will touch the figure of 400 million. Planning for this urban colossus is a herculean task. The shortages in housing, potable water and sanitation are already enormous and will grow further unless remedial action is taken in time. It does not, however, mean that all developmental activities must be halted or that we should go back to a simplistic life style. The provision of minimum needs of food, shelter, education and health to our vast masses demands that the basic industries and infrastructures such as agriculture, power, transport, communications, steel, fertilisers, pesticides, cement etc. be established.

One sees no option but to adopt the modern concepts of development, of course, after ensuring that these developmental patterns do not damage ecological balance as damage would not only hamper further development but also result in greater poverty for the poor who depend on the environment for food fuel, fodder and shelter. For the sustenance of a socio-political system aimed at people's welfare, protection of environment is as important as economic development. The two concepts are totally inter-dependent and form the essence of the concept of 'sustainable development'. Our country's ingenuity and creativity should, therefore, be directed towards identifying a developmental path which is harmony with environmental considerations.

The responsibility to harmonise environmental protection with development objectives rests with the Ministry of Environment and Forests. It serves as a focal point for the planning, promotion and coordination of various environmental and forestry programmes.

The task is sought to be fulfilled through action on diverse fronts such as survey and conservation of natural resources, impact assessment of development projects, incorporation of environmental protection in the planning process, control of pollution, regeneration programmes, legislation, research, extension, education, training, dissemination of information and creation of environmental awareness. The State Governments, Central and State Pollution Control Boards, the Indian Council of Forestry Research & Education, the Wildlife Institute of India, the Botanical and Zoological Survey of India and a host of other agencies are partners in the activities related to environment protection. A number of initiatives have been taken in the past few years to put environmental protection on firm ground.

Forest Conservation

Forests play an important role in maintaining environmental stability and in supplying the essential requirements of the people on a renewable basis. Over the years the forests have suffered depletion due to relentless pressures arising from the increasing demand for fuelwood, fodder and timber; inadequacy of protection measures; diversion of forestlands to non-forest uses, and the tendency to look upon forests as a revenue earning resource.

Realisation regarding importance of the forests has always been with us, but the first practical step came in the shape of the Forest Conservation Act, 1980 which prohibited diversion of forest lands for non-forest purposes, except with the previous permission of the Central Government. Under this Act, such permissions are generally refused. Where unavoidable for development purposes, permission is given only under condition of compensatory reforestation. This Act has been amended in 1988 to make the provisions more stringent and to enforce penalties even against officers who facilitate violation of this law. As a result of strict enforcement, the rate of diversion of forest land has been brought down to about 16,000 hectares per annum compared to the rate of 1.5 lakh hectares, per annum prior to this Act.

Other efforts to conserve forests include promotion of improved energy efficient stoves and alternative energy source. Modern forest fire control methods have already been adopted by some States to control forest fires. In 1985 the National Wastelands Development Board was set up to promote afforestation. The objective was to bring five million hectares of wasteland every year under fuelwood and fodder plantations with the participation of the people.

The Board has succeeded in afforesting 7.16 million hectares till the end of March 1989 through its programmes on social and agro forestry. While this achievement is substantial, the target of five million hectares per year is yet to be attained. In order to achieve the same, a comprehensive technology mission will be launched shortly. This technology mission will marshal the scientific and technological inputs available in our country to reclaim saline and alkaline lands and other kinds of wastelands to afforest the upper catchment areas of our important rivers and to meet the fuelwood and fodder requirements of the people.

Wildlife Conservation

The Wildlife (Protection) Act, 1972 has been amended to prohibit trade in endangered species and derivatives thereof. The National Wild life Action Plan has been implemented for a rational and modern wildlife management. A comprehensive report, "Planning and Wildlife Protected Area Network in India", has been prepared and released.

The scheme "Project Tiger" has been expanded for the maintenance of a viable population of the tigers in India, with 17 Tiger reserves in 13 States of the country covering an area of 26,643 sq.km.

National forest policy

The Natioanl Forest Policy adopted in 1952 aimed at forest coverage of one-third of the total land area of the country. But this could not be attained for various reasons and the process of deforestation continued. This has necessitated area-examination of the forest policy. The revised National Forest Policy was finalised after extensive consultation with the States, experts and all relevant agencies.

The salient feature of the new forest policy are: maintenance of environmental stability through preservation and restoration of ecological balance; conservation of the natural heritage of the country by preserving the remaining natural forests and protecting the vast genetic resources for the benefit of posterity; meeting the basic needs of the people, especially fuelwood, fodder and small timber for the rural and the tribal people and maintaining the intrinsic relationship between forests and the tribal and other poor people living in and around forests by protecting their customary rights and concessions on the forests.

Pollution control

India faces serious problems of environmental pollution. Water pollution from untreated community and industrial wastes flowing into our rivers and streams flowing into our rivers and streams, increasing use of fertilisers and pesticides, dumping of organic and inorganic wastes etc. are issues that need to be tackled on priority. Air pollution, long regarded as the bane of industrialised nations looms large over our country. The main instruments for control of pollution of water, air and noise are the Water (Prevention and Control of Pollution) Act, 1974, the Air (Prevention and Control of Pollution) Act, 1981, the Water Cess Act, 1977 and the Environment (Protection)Act, 1986.

The Water and Air Acts have been amended in the recent years to make provisions more stringent. The Pollution Control Boards have also taken up systematic monitoring of air and water quality through a network of quality monitoring stations-3.6 for water and 14 for air. Out of the nearly 4,000 major and medium polluting industries, more than half have already installed pollution control equipments. Standards have been notified for 26 priority industries. So far 3,300 prosecutions have been launched by the Pollution Control Boards against recalcitrant industries.

Ganga Action Plan

More than two-thirds of the pollution in our rivers is

caused by human and cattle wastes. In 1985 the Government took up a masssive project to clean up Ganga, the most important river of India. A Central Ganga Authority has been set up and an action plan was drawn up for cleaning the polluted stretches of the river Ganga by intercepting, diverting and treating about 900 mld. of the domestic waste water generated along the river to conform to effluent standards.

Schemes of low cost sanitaton, river front development, construction of electric crematoria etc. have keen taken up. Two hundred and sixty-two schemes have so far been sanctioned under the Ganga Action Plan at a cost of Rs.258.44 crore covering the States of Uttar Pradesh, Bihar and West Bengal. Fifty schemes have already been completed. Extensive awareness and public involvement activities have been taken up involving youth, students and pilgrims.

The Indian tradition of conservation can be traced back to pre-historic times. The theme of conservation prevades Indian culture, art and all its religions, Hindu, Muslim, Christian and Sikh. From Indira Gandhi's address to the Stockholm conference in 1972 to Rajiv Gandhi's address to the United Nations in 1988, and Environment Minister Shri Kamal Nath's address in Rio conference in 1992 India's leaders articulated the environmental concern of India effectively.

In India the last decade had seen the rise of public involvement. Silent Valley, the Doon Valley limestone quarries, the Chipko Movement, the protests against Narmada and Tehri...these mark a beginning. In response to them came a few legislative measures-the Environment Protection Act, the strengthening of the Air and Water Acts, the new Forest Policy...all these followed the creation of an environment ministry which started off as a lame duck waiting-room ministry for politicians and now, is being taken seriously. As the environmental problems have already reached an alarming situation. The concern for environment is felt by people all over the globe. Environmental Impact has become the focus of development programmes.

Response to Environmental Challenges

Environmental problems in India can be classified into two broad categories:

(a) Those arising from conditions of poverty and under development.

(b) Those arising as negative effects of the very process of development.

The first category has to do with the impact on the health and integrity of our natural resources (land, soil, water, forests, wild life, etc.) as a result of poverty and the inadequate availability, for a large section of our population, of the means to fulfil basic human needs (food, fuel, shelter, employment, etc).

The second category has to do with the unintended side-effects of efforts to achieve rapid economic growth and development. In this latter category would fall distortions imposed on national resources from poorly planned development projects and programmes, as from lack of attention to long-term concern by commercial and vested interests. Thus, it is clear that a concern for environment is essentially a desire to see that national development proceeds along rational sustainable lines. Environmental conservation is in fact the vary basis of all development. In India the over-riding concern for environment protection has been stressed in the Directive Principles of the Constitution of India.

To integrate the environmental concerns in the planning process, a high level National Committee on

Environmental Planning and Co-ordination (NCEPC) was set up in 1972.The Committee had done valuable work in a number of areas related to environmental planning. These include environmental appraisal of development projects, human settlements planning, formulation of environmental guidelines and creating environmental awareness at various levels. In the recognition of the need for a fresh comprehensive look at the administrative and legislative aspect of environmental protection, the Government of India constituted a High Power Committee under the Chairmanaship of the Deputy Chairman of the Planning Commission, Shri. N.D. Tiwari. The Tiwari Committee as this Committee is popularly known submitted its report to the Prime Minister in September, 1980.

National Environmental Advisory Committee

A National Environmental Advisory Committee was constituted in 1983 for highlighting environmental issues and giving advice on remedial action; raising public discussion on national issues of environmental significance, promoting public commitment and participation in environmental programmes, and providing feedback on people's perception of national environmental priorities and action plans.

Report of Tiwari Committee

The Tiwari Committee had identified the following major areas of environmental concern;

(a) *Environmental pollution*: All our rivers, lakes and ponds are heavily polluted by the discharge into them of untreated sewage and industrial effluents. The pollution constitutes a most dangerous health hazard apart from creating adverse effects on fish production and recreational possibilities, etc. It is also known that only a microscopic proportion of our industries are at present adequately treating their liquid effluents before discharging them into natural outfalls. The pollution of air by untreated gaseous effluents from industrial plants and by the exhausts of transport vehicles also constitutes a serious health hazard in many of our bigger towns.

Noise pollution has became a problem in many of our bigger towns.

(b) Land and Water resources: The mismanagement of our land and therefore also our water resources is of awesome scale. According to estimates made by Ministry of Agriculture in March 1980 as much as 175 million hectares (mh) out of the country's total land area of 304 mh, for which records exist, are subject to environmental problems.

In a study made in 1972, it was estimated that on an average, India was losing about 6000 million tonnes of top soil per annum through water erosion and that these represented in terms of major nutrients NPK alone, an annual loss of Rs. 700 crores. The corresponding loss today must be of a much higher order. Again, according to the Report of the National Commission on Floods (1980) the losses on account of floods average to over Rs. 100 crores per year. The total area subject to periodic floods which was estimated at 20 million hectares in 1971 now stands at the level of 40 million hectares.

Soil erosion also causes the premature siltation of tanks and reservoirs. The threat s of particular seriousness because in most cases of multi-purpose projects alternative sites for storage are just not available even if we can find the large sums of money needed to build new reservoirs in place of those which go out of commission.

The extent of forest cover is a good indicator of the health of the land. The large scale deforestation in recent decades had rendered the sensitive catchment areas in the Himalayan and other hilly areas particularly vulnerable to soil erosion. Poor land management thus aggravated the problems of droughts and floods.

No more than about 12 per cent of the country's land surface is actually under adequate tree cover as against the target of 33 per cent prescribed by the National Forest Policy of 1952. Further, although 13 million hectares are classed as "Permanent Pastures", these areas are in fact generally without any vegetation on account of either overgrazing or encroachments. Mention must also be made of the damage caused to our agricultural land in canal irrigated areas by water-logging and consequent salinisation on account of our failure to provide them with adequate drainage. It is estimated that about 6 million hectares of goodlands are affected by varying degrees of salinity.

The problems are so formidable in nature and scope that the Committee recommended "as a first step the setting up of Capital Land Commission" to look into issues concerning the health and scientific management of our total land resources.

(c) Natural Living Resources: With the inadequate level of scientifc knowledge in the country, it is not known how many species of flora and fauna are threatened, endangered or extinct; but it must be considerable considering the very rapid shrinkage of all natural forests and other ecosystems throughout the sub-continent in recent years.....The diversity of biological organisms a vital resource which needs to be carefully protected in natural ecosystems if we are not to close many possible evolutionary options for benefitting future generations. There is inadequate knowledge and understanding of our country's valuable marine ecosystems and total absence of protective measures has led to the wanton exploitation and destruction of these resources.

(d) Human settlements: It was not possible for the Committee, within the limited time available, to go into these aspects in any details. Therefore, it suggested that a separate group be constituted to study this subject area and its implifications for the environment.

However, the major problems of human settlements in India are well-known. Leaving aside the elitist residential and commercial areas in some of our bigger towns, the general condition of our human settlement is, to put it mildly, far from satisfactory from almost every point of view. While it would be futile to expect any significant improvement in these conditions for many years, and perhaps decades to come, there are two matters which we cannot afford to neglect any longer. These concern the indescribably poor sanitary conditions which prevail in almost all our villages and towns and our failure to supply clean drinking water to the vast majority of our people. Filth and dirt, and open drains and stinking sewage, along with the swarms of flies and mosquitoes which they breed, are to be seen everywhere. The supply of safe drinking water has become a problem even in our biggest towns, so much so that even cities like Delhi and Bombay are visited by epidemics of jaundice and other water-borne diseases every now and then.

(e) Environmental Awareness and Education: A sound, well-informed interest in nature among our people needs to be cultivated. Nature education, at all levels of education and public communication, must be efficiently organised especially in our schools.

New Legislative requirements

Some of the important legislative measures suggested by the Committee for recommending Legislative Measures and Administrative Machinery for ensuring environmental protection are as follows.

(i) Biosphere reserves: The Government may consider comprehensive legislation to give effect to the objectives to be served by Biosphere Reserves. Such legislation should include provisions for designating areas characterised by considerable genetic diversity in economic plants or are valuable for serving as "hot spot screening nurseries" for screening material for the detection of genes for resistance to pests as "Genesanctuaries".

(ii) Protection of Grazing Lands: The States be persuaded to enact suitable legislative support for the protection of Grazing Lands.

(iii) Protection of Endangered species: Supporting Indian legislation to effectively implement the Convention on International Trade in Endangered Species of Wild Fauna and Flora (CITES) to which India is a party.

(iv) Toxic Substances Control Act: This is required to ensure the protection of the environment from the sale manufacture, use and disposal of chemicals other than pesticides.

(v) Scientific Land Use: The existing regulations relating to the use of fertile soil for brick-making mining etc. require careful scrutiny. Suitable legislative provisions will have to be made to prevent the growing abuse of land and for enforcing strict reclamation regimes after the soil is removed for brick-making.

(vi) Prevention of noise pollution: Comprehensive legislation is required to cover the outdated bits and pieces of related unimplemented legislation at present on the statute books.

(vii) Prevention of denudation of forests: Legislative measures should be devised to curb the degradation caused by the greed of commercial interests through severe punishment while appropriate steps should be taken to meet the needs of those below the poverty line for fuel and fodder.

The Administrative Measures Suggested by Tiwari Committee

(i) The committee expressed the need for creating a Department of Environment (DOE) at the Centre under the charge of the Prime Minister to provide explicit recognition to the pivotal role that environmental conservation must play for sustainable national development. (The recommendation was accepted and a Department of the Environment duly constituted in 1980. The Department of Environment is the focal point within the Government of India for environmental management. The Department of Environment has, in addition to its catalytic promotional role in environmental management at the national level, executive functions in the field of pollution control. It also undertakes major programmes for ecological restoration.)

(ii) In order to conserve the nation's ecological base it was recommended that a Central Land Commission should be set up. (The recommendation has since been accepted by the Government and steps are being taken to implement it.)

(iii) Action taken to preserve/improve the environment.

The steps to preserve/improve the environment have been as follows:

(a) Pollution Control: The Central Board for Prevention and Control of Water Pollution (which is under the administrative control of the Department of Environment), together with the State Pollution Control Boards, completed a country-wide rapid inventory of pollution from large and medium industries. This was in execution of the "Control of Pollution at Source" programme. Minimal National Standards (MINAS) for polluting discharges from specific industries were formulated, and control measures implemented in a progressively stringent manner. About thirty percent of large and medium industries of the country have installed pollution control equipment.

A network of about 120 monitoring stations to check water pollution has been established. Zoning and classification of all the 14 major inter-state rivers have been completed to provide a basis for water quality management. The river basin-wise inventory for the Yamuna and Ganga has also been completed.

The Air Pollution Control Act became effective from May, 1981. Programmes in progress, after the framing and notification of rules under the Act completed, include strengthening of administrative support system, inventory of area to be declared air pollution control zones, evolution of ambient air quality standards as well as industry specific emission standard.

Projects in fields such as industry, energy, irrigation and mining have been subjected to environmental impact assessments, on the basis of information provided by the project authorites and supplemented by the Department of Environment's information gathering machinery.

(b) Land Resource Management: Notable efforts have been made to plan, organise and provide funds to improve desert environments. To improve ecology as also to meet the requirements of the local cattle and human population forestry has been taken up relatively extensively. Rural electrification with a view to assisting the exploitation of ground water has been promoted. Construction of Rajasthan Canal envisages to transform barrren un-inhabited areas of western Rajasthan into a vast granary. With a view to meeting the basic and economic needs of the community, the programme of

Social Forestry-which inter alia includes Farm Forestry. Extension Forestry Reforestation in degraded forests and Recreation Forestry-to augment the supply of fuel wood, fodder and small timber to rural areas was taken up in the Sixth Plan to cover 100 chronically deficit districts.

The new 20-points Economic Programme of the late Prime Minister included afforestation, social forestry and farm forestry. A National Eco-Development Board has been set up to achieve sustainable eeconomic and social development through national utilization of natural resources-water, soil , plant and animal life.

In order to demonstrate methodologies for reclamation of environmentally degraded areas, to create general environmental awareness and to involve public participation in the solution of environmental problems a number of projects have been carried out by the Department of Environment under its Eco-Development Programme.

Universities in several States and voluntary agencies organised Eco-Development Camps. Task Forces of ex-service personnel for eco-developmental work in Shivaliks (UP), Rajasthan Canal etc. have been raised. Programmes have also been formulated for extension of eco-developmental work for mined area reclamation, environment in metropolitan settlements, hill resorts, pilgrimage centres and the Himalayan foothills, etc.

(c) Natural living resources: India has initiated the formulation of a National Conservation Strategy. It has also adopted a National Wild Life Action plan during the year 1983-84, 13 sites in different biographical regions have been identifed for designation as Biosphere Reserves. Work on environmental impact assessment, wildlife conservation and faunal composition of different eco-systems has been taken up. Studies on faunal composition of marine, estuarine, fresh water and terrestrial eco-systems have been conducted in some areas. Activities to survey, identify and investigate plant species are underprogress. The Botanical Survey of India (BSI) has set up a countrywide network with regional offices. The herbaria of the survey hold over 2 million plant specimens. More than 150 new plants have been discovered.

Survey of unexplored areas, intensification of the District Flora Programme, preparation of comprehensive documents on new flora of India and study of endemic and treated plants were among the major programmes. It has also been involved in assessment of environmental impact of several developmental projects and inventorisation of plant resources in important eco-systems. These include the Silent Valley, Sutlej-Beas Link, Tehri Dam, Lalpur Dam, Idukki Valley etc. and National Parks. Games sanctuaries and areas to be designated as Biosphere Reserves.

The Zoological Survey of India has primarily been engaged in the survey of faunal resources and collection of base-line scientific data with regard to their taxonomy bio-ecology animal behaviour and pollution, etc. Special emphasis was given to the studies on the ecology and population of rare and endangered animals and birds. Studies on final composition of marine, estuarine, fresh water and terrestrial eco-systems were conducted.

(d) Environmental Awareness: Programmes have been addressed to specific target groups such as planners and decision-makers, administrators, executives, students, etc. For higher level administrators, senior executives and planners a series of carefully structured workshops were organised at the Administrative Staff College of India, Hyderabad, the Indian Institute of Management, Bangalore and the Indian Institute of Public Administration, New Delhi. To generate environmental awareness in the public, nation-wide celebrations of World Environment Day and Wildlife Week are organised every year. The first National Environmental Congress and first National Conference of Legislators on Environment have also been held. The National Museum of National History (NMNH) further expanded its facilities for non-formal environmental education, and catered to wide spectrum of the public with particular emphasis on children, and the disadvantaged and handicapped segments of society, in coordination with the States and Union Territories.

(e) Promotion of Environmental Research: Promotion of research has been one of the major activities aimed at developing information on various aspects of environmental management and for building up of scientific manpower to deal with the environmental problems. The projects are conducted by a number of universities, R&D institutions, non-governmental agencies and field formations of the Department of Environment. Monitoring of environmental parameters, pollution control, energy use, environmental aspects in human settlements, instrumentation, effects of pesticides and impact human activities on natural eco-systems are among the subject areas dealt with in such projects.

A distinctive feature in the research programme was the introduction of coordinated research projects in selected issues of national importance. These include an All India Coordinated Project on Heavy Metal, a multi-disciplinary project of Microbial Degradation of Industrial Waters, a coordinated project on Ethnobiology and multi-disciplinary studies for monitoring of environmental effects of the Idukki River Valley Project and Beas Sutlej link. In addition, under the Integrated Eco-Development Programme, action-oriented projects on identified priority areas have also been launched in the Himalayan Region, Western Ghats and the Ganga Basin.

As part of its programme to create a strong research base and training support, a number of centres of excellence are being set up. One such Centre for Ecological Research and Training with particular reference to the problems of the Western Ghats region has been set up at the Indian Institute of Science, Bangalore. An Institute on Himalayan Environment and Development is also in the process of being set up.

(f) Environmental Impact Assessment and Monitoring: Environmental appraisal is an important responsibility assigned to the Department of Environment. This involves evaluation of environment implications and incorporation of necessary safeguards for such activities having a bearing on environmental quality. Questionnaires for eliciting information on environmental aspects of development projects in selected sectors, such as industry, multipurpose river valley schemes, thermal power generation, shipping and harbours, and mining have been prepared. The project authorities are required to incorporate a chapter on environmental aspects in their feasibility reports.

(g) Centres of Excellence: Strengthening active research training groups in universities/institutions working in areas of interest is necessary. The Department of Environment proposes to selectively support such groups in priority areas of environmental science and management, such as mangrove ecosystem, environmental education, mine environment studies, etc.

The Ecological Research and Training Centre is one such centre already functioning at the Indian Institute of Science, Bangalore, where two scientific programmes have been initiated, viz., one on ecological science focusing on eco-development-oriented research on the Western Ghats and another on environmental studies programme focusing on training with special reference to air and water pollution.

(h) Environmental Information: The scheme for setting up of the Environmental Information System (ENVIS) with national network of Distributed Information Centres (DIC) and a focal point in the Department of Environment was approved in the Sixth Plan period. It has become operational through the installation of a Computer Terminal linked with the computer system of the National Informatics Centre (NIC) to serve as the focal point facility for storage, retrieval and dissemination of information to the users. Distributed Information Centres were set up at the Industrial Toxicology Research Centre, Lucknow, the Central Board for Prevention and Control of Water Pollution, New Delhi and 7 other centres for information services in specific subject areas. Centres in respect of other subject areas are being set up.

(i) Pitambar Pant National Environment Fellowship: The Pitambar Pant National Environment Fellowship Award was constituted by the Government of India in 1978 to encourage and recognise excellence in any branch or research related to the environmental sciences. The fellowship is awarded every year on the World Environment Day, i.e. on June 5. The fellowship is in recognition of significantly important research/ development contri-bution and is also intended to encourage talented individuals to devote themselves whole time to R & D pursuits in the field of environmental sciences for the duration of the fellowship, which is two years.

International Cooperation and Legislation for Environmental Protection

(i) International Cooperation

In the period between the 1972 United Nations Conference on the Human Environment and now, the environment has moved into the mainstream of issues that concern the international community. In the UNEP

Government Council, and its numerous other areas, nations have found that they could reach a broad consensus on nature, magnitude and importance of international problems and measures needed to tackle them. Countries have a stake in each other's environmental welfare and stability. There is a massive scope without any impairment of sovereignty and countries legitimate rights for cooperative action on sound management of national resources. Agreement is already present between various groups of governments on a wide range of environmental issues. There is a perception of mutual benefits, UNEP's Regional Seas Agreements, the World Soils Policy, the draft Convention on the Protection of the Ozone Layer, the Trade in Endangered, Species, Wetlands and World Heritage Conventions between and among developed and developing countries are only a few examples. There are 113 conventions and protocols listed in UNEP's register of international treaties and other agreements in the field of the environment.

The principal focus for the dialogue on environment among developing nations has been the meetings of the non-aligned countries and the Group of 77. The UNEP Governing Council itself has provided a major forum for co-operation among the members of the Group of 77. Typical of the Governing Councils the prevailing spirit of cooperation is the provisions of US 1 million dollar by the Government of Argentina-to be used through UNEP's catalytic role-for technical assistance to help developing nations address serious environmental problems. Outside the Governing Council the South Asian Cooperative Environment Programme provides another example of mutual assistance among developing countries.

For the significant part of the last decade, the dialogue among developed countries focused largely on environmental pollution control provides an example.

But in recent years there has been a marked shift to adopting preventive policies and taking preventive measures. Notable achievement have included the adoption of the Convention on Long-Range Trans-boundary Air Pollution and OECD's guiding principles concerning international aspects of environmental policies and recommendations and decisions concerning the export and import of banned or severely restricted chemicals.

The decade since Stockholm has also witnessed an increase in environmental cooperation among the nations of the Council for Mutual Economic Assistance (CMEA). This has been accompanied by an increasing emphasis on environmental protection in the cooperation between CMEA Member States and developing countries which has included such topics as hydropower, water and land management and assistance with the installation of environmentally sound new plant and machinery.

Environmental issue may need to be dealt with on different geographical scales, as well as on different time-scales. In other words, they may arise, and/or require action, at the global, regional, sub-regional or other levels. Problems of global concern, including those of the joint management of the global commons and of environmental interdependence, can be dealt with in the overall setting of multilateral internaional negotiations. A case in point is the lay of the sea. There are also clearly identifiable issues characteristic of given geographical settings and countries, which are best dealt with regionally, sub-regionally or nationally, even though many of these have a broader significance.

(ii) National legislation

Since early 1970s there has been a massive expansion in the establishment of national environmental bodies (agencies, departments, councils, committees etc.). There has been considerable increase in the number of governmental and non-governmental bodies dealing with environmental issues. It is estimated that there was about 2,500 non-governmental organisations in 1972, the number rose to about 15,000 in 1981. The period saw also bursting legislation dealing with environmental issues both in developed and developing countries. In OECD nations, for example, whereas the 4 major national environmental laws were passed in 5 years 1956-60, 10 in 1961-65 and 18 in 1966-70, between 1971-1975, 31 such measures were adopted. and a further 25 followed in the 4 years 1976-79 inclusive. By the end of the 1970s statistics of reports on the state of the environment (or both) were being produced in many countries (for example, Germany, Federal Republic of Finland, Japan, Philippines, Spain, Sweden, United States of America).

(iii) Public Participation

The Stockholm Conference provided on impetus renewed interest in environmental education during the 1970s. In response to the Stockholm Recommendations, UNESCO and UNEP set up an International Environmental Education Programme which aims at promoting exchange of information and experiences in the field of environmental education.

Public participation in environmental affairs has increased. Some of the interest was spurred by the efforts of the media to cover the field.

Environmental awareness increased most in wealthier and better educated populations and stimulated by books and films as well as newspapers, magazines and the electronic media/ Non-governmental organisations played an important role in the development of a better understanding of environmental issue. Public organisations affected the decision-making process in a number of countries, particularly in connection with nuclear power development. On the whole, progress was apparent in both environmental education and public awareness of environmental issues during the decade.

(iv) Position in India

International Cooperation

India's Department of Environment functions as the nodal agency for United National Environment Programme (UNEP), the South Asia Cooperation Environment Programme (SACEP) and the International Union for Conservation of Nature and Natural Resource (IUCN). India has been actively participating in the various sessions of UNEP with a view to ensure that programmes are more relevant to the developing countries. The South Asia Cooperative Environment Programme has recently set up the inter-governmental organization with Afghanistan, Bangladesh, Butan, India, Maldives, Pakistan, Sri Lanka and Iran as its members. At the 1981 ministerial level meeting, areas were identified for implementation.

India was assigned the focal point responsibilities in the areas of Environment Education, Environmental Legislation and Wild Life Management. At the 1983 Government Meeting of SACEP number of projects have been identified for implementation in the area of Energy, Environmental Education, Legislation and Environmental Impact Assessment. India has a number of on-going Bilateral Programmes with both developed and developing countries.

INDEX